M000247808

Diary of Linda Woodall Salmons Swann

IN GOD WE TRUST

Linda Swann

ISBN 978-1-0980-4534-0 (paperback)
ISBN 978-1-0980-4535-7 (hardcover)
ISBN 978-1-0980-4536-4 (digital)

Copyright © 2020 by Linda Swann

All rights reserved. No part of this publication may be reproduced, distributed, or transmitted in any form or by any means, including photocopying, recording, or other electronic or mechanical methods without the prior written permission of the publisher. For permission requests, solicit the publisher via the address below.

Christian Faith Publishing, Inc.
832 Park Avenue
Meadville, PA 16335
www.christianfaithpublishing.com

Printed in the United States of America

In Remembrance of
Jeffrey Lee Salmons
4-15-1970 to 8-25-1989

I also want to thank my daughter, Anita,
for always being there.

About the Author

✝

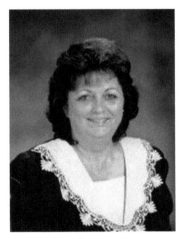

Linda Salmons Swann

Linda still lives in her hometown of Hamlin, West Virginia. Linda and Bob were married April 15, 1992. Bob passed away on April 29, 2020 after a long illness. They continued serving the Lord and attending Pleasant Hill Missionary Baptist Church where she has played the piano since she was thirteen years old. When Bob came into the church, he became the choir director, and together they have served the Lord.

During all those five years of Jeff's illness, they had much love and support from many friends, family, and community. Besides their family and friends a special thanks needs to be given to Linda's neighbor, Fay Weaver, who was always so willing to help!

The Lord blessed Linda and Bob with six grandchildren. Anita married Billy Edmonds, Jr. in 1990. Billy adopted Heather Lakin in 1992. They then had Lindsay Brooke in 1992 and Megan Lee in 1994. Billy, Anita and Lindsay have a gospel group, The Edmonds Family. Lakin, Lindsay and Megan all three serve the Lord. They are also graduates of Marshall University and work in fields helping others. Lakin Edmonds Donahue has one daughter, Meredith Lane. Lindsay is married to Patrick Lovejoy, who brought to the family Madalyn and Parker and together, they have Maggie Blair. Bob's daughter Tammy married Chris Bragg and they have three children, Tori, Aaron, and Tate. Tori has two children, a daughter, Jolea, and a son, Trapper. Aaron has one son, Trae.

Linda and Bob's home has been filled with love and blessings from God. Linda has always been very busy with work, church, family, taking care of her parents and sisters and a whole lot of little ones. Linda looks to God and thanks Him for these blessings and is still able to say, "*In God We Trust!*"

"God is our refuge and strength, a very present help in time of trouble." (Psalm 46:1)

Monday
December 31, 1984

Well it's New Year's Eve 1984. I haven't had or kept a diary since I was a teenager. Jeff and I are in Rockville, Maryland in a motel (Colonial Manor) away from all our family and my daughter. Jeff is not feeling very well. His counts are low.

I would have to go back several months for you to understand why we are here. Maybe, I'll start from years ago.

You know, I married Jack Salmons when I was nineteen, December 23, 1966. He was in college; I was working at the welfare office as a receptionist. I was very happy.

Well, after a couple of years, Anita was born November 5, 1968. Seventeen months later, Jeffrey was born April 15, 1970. They are two of the most beautiful and kind children in the world. Time just seemed to fly by—working, home, husband, children, and church. I was very happy. The Lord has been so good to us. When I look back now, I wonder why I was so happy, and seemingly after everything that has happened, Jack was not. I wonder if he were ever happy. You know, Jack quit going to church, and as time went by, he was never home. It seemed he couldn't enjoy home and playing with the kids. They used to want to play games and wrestle, rough house, but Jack was not a happy person, always searching for something.

Well, 1983, September, Labor Day, Jack decided he wanted another life, which did not include me.

Oh, he said he would still be the kid's father. He hardly ever called them. He asked Columbia Gas for a transfer to Houston, Texas. He said he couldn't face all the people around Hamlin.

You know, I had complete trust and faith in Jack in our marriage until the last few months before September 1983. How could I have been so wrong about Jack, the person, his moral values. Boy, did he ever fool me.

After Jack left, I found out a lot of things. Life wasn't so simple anymore. Not just black or white—right or wrong. I found myself married to a man who evidently made a pass at every woman he got the opportunity, whether it be a friend, a next-door neighbor, or even a sister and sister-in-law.

I tried to get Jack to get counseling. He said he didn't have a problem, but the fact remains *we* have a problem. I said for better or for worse and I meant that. Jack just seemed bent on throwing everything away. I really feel he found someone else, maybe someone he liked to socialize and party with. I can't drink and party like that. There is something inside, the Holy Spirit, dwelling there, directing my life. I've prayed for Jack for a long time. I don't know why he wanted away from everything.

He, at one time believed. He left with the words "I don't believe in nothing or nobody. I just want to exist. I can't pray." What happened to him?

You know, I never knew quite how to deal with Jack; it was hard for me to request prayer for him at church. Jack convinced me everything was all right. I guess I saw him the way I wanted to see him.

I always thought Jack and I had a good relationship, and plus, we loved each other, I thought. Up until the last year, things, I guess, just had to come up front—the truth always comes out. I guess Jack thought he had it covered and that it would never surface.

Jack stayed gone seven or eight years working on the ambulance service, and then when that folded, it became his job, or so I thought. I wonder how Jack really feels. I think if he did not have so much pride and I believe blinded by sin, the real person Jack is so different. When sin compounds, it begins to eat away at the very inner being of a person.

I was so hurt by all that has happened. I wonder how I, my children, have made it. But, we know the Lord was with us. I thought it was the worst thing ever, hurt, divorce. I still feel that I love Jack, but something is gone, and I guess that is trust. That feeling only two people in love can know. It's gone. It seems it meant nothing to Jack. He just used me, and when that wasn't enough shame and hurt, he just walked away, hurting not only the one who loved him the most but also two beautiful children. The sad thing is they had already lost faith in their father before he left, and I couldn't see it either.

Well, that trauma came and went. On February 14, I went before the judge. Divorce was granted, and you know Anita and Jeff begged me to divorce Jack. Do you think I did the wrong thing? I've prayed and read my Bible. I felt that it had to be done. I don't know, maybe Jack would never see what he gave up until it was gone.

I felt if he wanted out—did not want me or the kids—then I would give him his wish. Set him free. The Lord gave me and the kids strength to see us through. It brought us closer to Him and maybe felt a closer love. How could Jack have walked away from those who loved him?

Well, time went on—spring came and went. Summer came, off to the beach we went. That's what Anita and Jeff wanted. And you know what? Jeff sat out on the deck and looked out over the ocean, almost every night. What was he thinking? About the father that left or the pain? I know now, he may have been hurting more than we'll ever know.

You see, 1984, also brought another trauma to our lives. My son, that I love more than life itself, had cancer, and my daughter, who I also love more than life itself, is suffering heartache. We hurt for Jeff, who suffers physically in pain with this terrible disease. I ask myself, how could this be happening? He was playing football, weighed 188 pounds. Oh, he loved it so much. But he hurt so bad.

After surgery and the diagnosis, I couldn't believe it. Shock, a hurt that went to the very center of my very being. I want to hurt for him, take away the pain, but I can't. I can only pray, pray to the same God that has always been with us. He said he would never leave us. You know, it goes through my mind that maybe God has allowed this to happen for Jack to see, pray, turn himself around. But I try not to question it, only believe.

I believe in a God that has all power; nothing can happen to us that God cannot control. I ask for strength, so I can help Jeff. But you know "quiet" Jeff never ceases to surprise me. He is so wise for a fourteen-year-old. Once on the plane, we were looking at the clouds, he said, "Mom, someday we are going to walk on those suckers."

I said, "But Jeff we're going to walk on streets of gold."

He said, "Yeah but we have to come right up through here." Praise the Lord, my heart sings. Even in the midst of this hurt and suffering, his faith shines on. He also said in the hospital, "If I die, I'm going to that good place. I don't know about Dad."

Oh, if Jack could only see. How could he walk away and not be with his beautiful children? Anita also has suffered so much hurt, but she too, knows where to take her cares, the Lord and Savior Jesus Christ. She even made her way down the aisle at our little church to pray for her father. Oh, Jack, what you gave up! How many fathers and mothers have and will pray for two such children.

They're yours, Lord, and my life also. But sometimes, I feel like I don't do too good in living my Christian life. It seems I don't know what to say sometimes, but I do pray that my life will mean something for the Lord.

Jeff has a lot of tough treatment to go, but I feel in my heart a plan being worked out. You know, I believe in prayer and the One to whom we pray. I believe He has the power to touch Jeff and feel that He already has. Praise the Lord, Satan can and will be defeated. He's trying so hard to pull us down.

"Lord, I pray for strength through this, to be with Jeff, ease his pain, strengthen him physically, spiritually, and emotionally." If it takes the treatment and us being here in Maryland (National Cancer Institute), away from home, then we will trust in God, and he will have the best treatment possible. I feel the Lord worked it out for us to come here.

We miss Anita so much. You know how hard it must be, but she says whatever it takes for Jeff to get well, she can manage. She has been left with no father at home, her mother, and her brother in a faraway place. Oh, I love her so much, too. I think she knows that. Thank the Lord for family and friends.

Well, that brings us up to New Year's Eve, 1984, tonight, in a motel in Maryland.

What will 1985 hold?

Well, the Bible says, "Not to worry what tomorrow may bring. God will provide!" In Him, we have anchored our faith. My mind wonders to our little church, Pleasant Hill, our family, friends seated there right now, worshipping in Spirit and Truth. What a blessing! I know they are praying for us too. The next page will bring in a new year.

"In God, We Trust!"

✝

Tuesday
January 1, 1985

Well, we're in the hospital at NIH. At midnight last night, Jeff and I sat in the lobby of the Colonial Manor Motel, waiting for a cab to take us to the hospital. The New Year came, and we rode to the hospital. During the ride, my heart ached, and tears came to fill my eyes. Jeff felt so bad, and my heart ached for him. The cab driver said, "Happy New Year." I said "1984 has not been very good and I hope 1985 will be better." He said he felt the same way and hoped so too.

So, we are here, Jeff is getting antibiotics, IV, and blood transfusion right now. It's 7:30 p.m. We've talked to Anita, Wanda, Mother and Mrs. Salmons. Jack called a little while ago; he didn't even bother to call and talk to Jeff on New Year's Eve or Anita either. I can hardly stand to talk to him anyway. I don't want to hate, and I can pray for him, but it just makes me sick and angry when I really think about what Jack has done. Most of the time, I just try to push everything to the back of my mind. If I really think about it, I just could go to pieces. A woman up here at the hospital told me she heard him on the phone telling someone how much he loved her and missed her. That just about did it for me. How much more can it hurt? I don't know.

But I do know I have to let go. I guess I'll always pray for Jack, but I guess I can only deal with it by turning the burden over to the Lord. I just don't know what else to do.

I wonder about life since all this has happened. I think I've really learned what the word *faith* means. I've read about it and believed in it, but we are actually, truly living each day by faith.

Faith, it seems to me, is just learning and trusting in the Lord's promises.

There are many promises to be found in His Holy Word. We must not lose sight of the promise. There is so much suffering at the hospital, young people, and children. Oh, the curse of this sinful world. Someday, it will not be like this. Everything will be new; old things will pass away, no more suffering, no more heartache, no more tears! Read Revelation. Oh, such sweet promises to His children.

O God, please, give us strength each and every day. We can't make it alone, and O God, sometimes I do feel so all alone. Thank God for His marvelous peace and love.

Well, I have to go now. It's almost eight, and Jeff and I are having peanut butter and crackers. I'm so glad he's eating something. I pray to the Lord to be with us through the night.

"In God We Trust!"

✝

Wednesday
January 2, 1985

Well, we've spent another day at NIH. Jeff had radiation simulation today. They drew lines on his hip. Tomorrow, he has a CT scan, and Friday, he has more lines drawn on him for radiation.

Jack called this morning; I could hardly talk to him. He calls and says, "How are you?" It seems such a mockery for him to ask how I am, what does he care? I just can't react to that. The real concern and love that I need to feel just doesn't come from Jack. Jeff was asleep, and I was finally at the point of tears. I told him I just didn't feel like talking to him at all.

Forgive me, Lord.

I try to be as kind and considerate as I can. There's just so much hurt there. But I do pray for Jack; he needs the Lord. How can he be happy and not want to live what he knows to be right?

Dr. Arndt came in this evening and told us that the bone marrow and bone biopsy in Jeff's left pelvic was *negative!* Praise the Lord!

Dr. Arndt was surprised. Jeff said, "I wasn't." You know, again quiet Jeff surprises me. I feel Jeff has, deep inside, a very strong faith. Praise the Lord! They didn't expect it to be negative this quickly. Matthew 8, I believe Jesus said, "I will come and heal him."

I believe those words were not only for the days that Jesus actually walked on this earth; they are for today and always.

Jesus has all the *power* given to him by the eternal father. Praise the Lord! We pray for the strength for the tough treatment that is to follow.

Jack called again; I pray that I can deal with this. The resentment just builds inside. I pray for forgiveness and pray that I can forgive Jack for all the hurt he has caused in our lives.

But right now, we just want to thank God for His healing hand and the peace He's given us deep inside. Anita called too. Love her heart, she was so excited. She said tell me everything. Anita needed that too. She said it really cheered her up.

"Oh God, I pray we can live for His glory. You know I feel it won't be very long until he comes back for his children. I thank Him for a special day and the good news, that we know came from Heaven, although Dr. Arndt maybe thinks she did, Dr. Arndt was the messenger. I wonder if she knows that."

"In God We Trust!"

✝

Saturday
January 5, 1985

Boy, it's Saturday. Time does pass. Sometimes you think it will not pass. You sit here for about seven days and nights, and sometimes, I get this feeling inside. I don't know how to explain it, nervousness, anxiety, or something. But I have to control it, or I'll fall apart, and Jeff needs me too much for that. Sometimes though, we both cry. If he cries, I cry. You know, it seems to help, I guess. I tell Jeff we're just putting our faith in the Lord God Almighty, and the Lord gives us an inner peace. We *cannot* make it without Him. We know that. Anita calls us faithfully two or three times a day. Oh, we miss her so much. She's going to try and come spend a week with us later in January.

Jeff is feeling a little better. His fever stayed down last night. The doctor started him on another antibiotic, which makes four because of his gums. His urine was also getting concentrated a lot and burning him.

You know, I feel there is a reason for all this. I don't know exactly what, and you know a person could become very bitter. You think, why your child? But I guess like Jeff said, "Why anybody?" Someday, we'll understand. I long for that day when Jesus will come and stop all this suffering. Then Satan will have no more power. Christ will reign as King. But I feel there is a lot of work to do on this earth. So many unsaved people that needs to find the Lord. Maybe this will touch someone, Jeff's suffering. Jeff is quiet most of the time, but I feel someday, (in my heart, I feel the Lord has something in store for Jeff to do), he will have a lot to say. Let us not forget about this suffering, of all these children.

"Oh, I pray to God, a cure for this dreadful disease will be found. Please Lord, I pray."

Well, I'm going to read my Bible now. I started on the New Testament when we first started coming up here. I have found the time to read. I've read so much, and Christ did so much healing when He was on this earth and I didn't seem to realize how many instances are recorded in the Bible. God has all the power, and I believe deep in my heart and I know Jeff believes, too, that Christ will see him through this and has already touched his body. Praise the Lord!

"For whatever reason we are here, I pray for strength for us all, Jeff, me, Anita and those back home. I do pray for Jack. He needs the Lord. Help me forgive Lord and accept your will in my life."

*****

Sunday

We're back in the motel. We got here about three-thirty. I walked to the store and got a few groceries and washed dishes. Jeff and I put a magazine rack together. He sanded it and painted it.

I went down to the dining room and ate a salad. Jeff just wanted a bologna and cheese sandwich. We've watched TV, and Jeff is reading a book I bought him.

Roger, a high school friend, called twice today. You know, he wants us all to go to the beach with him and his children; I'm not sure about this. I think maybe Roger is looking for a serious relationship, and I cannot even get past friendship right now. I enjoy him coming up. Anita and Jeff enjoy his children coming up too. But I don't love Roger. I can't seem to let go of seventeen years of marriage. Sometimes, I hurt so bad I just don't know what I feel. I think I still love Jack, and oh, how much I've wanted to forgive Jack, but he's never asked. And how many times I just wanted to say, "I love you Jack, let's try and work things out," but Jack is not interested at all. I just don't understand. I loved him so much, and I thought he loved me. How could I have been so wrong? Now Jack is living with some woman down in Texas. How could this have ever happened? Jack betrayed me and the kids. A lot of time I really get angry and have a hard time even talking to him. I don't know. I pray and pray and sometimes I think I ask God for too much, but I pray to the One, God Almighty. Nothing is impossible with Him. I pray for a Christian home with Jack, me, and the kids serving God, and the healing hand of God to touch Jeff. Satan tells me you can't expect God to do all that, but I feel in my heart still that all this is possible. God answers prayers and we love Him. And, in Him we have put our trust.

Jeff is feeling pretty good. He always says he's tired. He said he has been tired ever since he had the surgery on December 17, 1984. We talked to Anita today too. We miss her so much.

In God We Trust.

*****

Tuesday

Well, another day has passed. Jeff had more radiation today. Tomorrow after radiation, Jeff sees the doctor in radiation, and I'm glad because I have some questions.

He's eating peanut butter and crackers now, doing homework and watching A-Team.

Anita called; she's gone to the Hamlin and GV game. She plays in the Pep band with her piccolo. Anita seems real excited about coming out to stay.

Jack called this evening. He said he wants to call every day or every other day to see how we are, and he says, "Hang in there." I just cannot do anything but answer his questions. Jack has never been around when we need him. How does he really feel? Only God knows. I wonder what kind of relationship Jack has with this other woman? Does he love her? Did he love all the others? Or was it just a way of life Jack thought he wanted or found out he could make passes. Why did he have to prove he could or was that what he was doing? I don't know, I just don't know. Jack has never been able to tell me anything that would make things clearer, other than he says he has changed. Boy, that is an understatement!

What is wrong with me? Jack and I, I thought, had a special kind of love, an everlasting love, even when Jack returned no love to me. When we didn't have much money, had debts, and sickness, I never stopped loving Jack, and now after everything, I still love him. Is that possible and if so, I don't know about the future. This is where I have to turn to the Lord. I don't know what the future holds, but I know who holds the future. That is the peace I feel inside. A future without Jack, I don't know. At times, I think "Linda okay, Jack is living with another woman, we are divorced. It's over, and other people say you are better off." But I don't feel that way, and maybe I should. But how do you quit loving someone so easily? What will the future hold? *In God We Trust.* That's all I know and believe. Jack says he believes with his mouth but where is his heart? Only God knows, his life does not bear witness, but only God can judge.

I pray to God to forgive him. Jack let his life get out of hand, and I don't want him to be lost. I love him, and I ask God to forgive him.

Well, Jeff is still working on homework, and we're watching A-Team.

Sometimes, I feel anxiety and worry, and I think it will take me over, and then, I have to pray for strength.

Please Lord see us through this and then I know the answer. He will!

"In God We Trust!"

*****

Thursday

Well, we are in the hospital. Jeff is getting chemo today and tomorrow. It's 10:30 p.m. He hasn't got sick yet, but usually, it takes four hours. Maybe he won't get as sick this time. I hope not. He's reading the Battle of the Bulge now.

Wanda, David, Davy, and Anita are coming up tomorrow. Anita is going to stay all next week with us. We miss her so much!

They put us on the third floor this time in a private room because there is no room on the sixth floor. It sure is quieter here.

I read a book by Hal Lindsey today called *The Rapture*. It thrills my heart to read about the rapture of the Church. You know, I don't think it will be very long before the Lord takes his children away. "Snatches" us away as Hal Lindsey calls it. Oh, what a glorious promise.

Thank you, Lord, for the feeling deep inside that excites our very inner being. We're going home soon to suffer no more. But my heart aches for the unsaved, so many. I pray to live a life that I might lead souls to God. I pray for my children, that they will always live for the Lord. Because I know that is the most important thing. I ask God for strength to help us through the night and be with Jeff. We need the Lord so much and ask Him to give the family a safe trip up tomorrow.

"In God We Trust"

✝

Sunday
January 13, 1985

Well, we're beginning another week of radiation treatment. Jeff just had chemo for two days, and he didn't get quite as sick this time. We thank the Lord!

Anita is here with us now; it is so good her being here with us. We have missed her so much. Jeff really likes her being here. Wanda, David, and Davy called back they got home about 7:00 p.m. I really appreciate them coming.

Sometimes, I think I'm going to break down when everyone is here, but I try not to. Sometimes, I feel everyone is on the verge of tears. It hurts so much. I think we all hurt for Jeff. But the Lord always gives us strength. We can feel the prayers of everyone, our friends, family, church family, everyone. We thank God for that help. We believe in prayers; we believe in the One to whom we pray!

Anita and Jeff have worked on some homework, taken a nap, watched TV, and now they're going to go play a video game here in the motel lobby in the minute.

Jeff has five more weeks of radiation to go. I have to admit I get a feeling in the pit of my stomach when I think of the next weeks and months. I get nervous, nauseous, homesick, scared, and lonely and worried all together. But all I can do is ask the Lord to be with us and lean on him.

I don't understand any of this, Jack, Jeff's illness, and sometimes life itself. If I didn't have the Lord to turn to, where could I go?

"I ask God to help Jeff, now through this treatment and in the future to deal with everything. I guess that worry will always be there, Cancer. I sometimes wonder if we'll ever really recover from all this, and I guess really be happy again. But I'm trusting in the Lord, and I pray Anita and Jeff will always be faithful to the Lord and put their trust in him."

"In God We Trust"

Saturday
January 19, 1985

Well, a week has passed since I wrote in the diary. Anita went home today. The week passed so quickly. I miss Anita so much, but she had to get back in school, and this is Jeff's fever period. If he goes in the hospital, she wouldn't have anywhere to stay. Anita's life has been turned upside down too. I pray for her that she will keep her faith and lean on the Lord. We are trusting in the Lord. We love the Lord. He wants us to be happy, Jeff to be well and Jack serving him, and you know what, God has the power to answer those prayers. We need to exercise our faith; I believe God has all power. You know when you really stop and think of who you're serving it is really almost overwhelming, the power, as close as prayers.

"O, Heavenly Father, help us to pray, really pray in faith in God believing. Thank you, Lord. Praise the Lord, for your beautiful promises. I believe the Lord has already touched Jeff, and God will see him through this. There are great things ahead for Jeff, Anita, and us as a family. I can feel it deep down inside. We're serving a Great God!"

Praise the Lord!
Thank the Lord!
"In God We Trust"

†

Well, we are in the hospital. Jeff has a fever and is not feeling too well.

He got Johnny Toppings as a roommate. He's from Hurricane, West Virginia and we've got to be friends with Johnny and his mom, Linda. She is also divorced and remarried to Roger Horn, and has two children by him, Tammy (fifteen) and Roger (ten). Sort of funny isn't it?

I was hoping Jeff would not get a fever this time, but we are here. We just have to deal with it. At one last night he got sick. I had to load everything up and heat my car. It was four this morning before we got to bed. I forgot some groceries and had to go back to the motel and get them. I went on up to McDonald's and got me a Big Mac. I was so hungry; it seemed funny being by myself. I have a king size headache. I guess because of no sleep.

Last night, we went down to chest X-ray. I stood and watched Jeff. It just breaks my heart to see him suffer, but Jeff's suffering will turn in to happiness, tears to a smile, and heartache into joy because he loves the Lord. The Lord is so good. Thank you, Lord, for being with us, the healing hand and marvelous love and promises. I really need the Lord's help. Please, I am so weak, but he is strong. I ask the Lord to be with Anita too. Give her strength and courage and wrap her in His love.

"In God We Trust"

✝

Monday
January 28, 1985

Well, Jeff got out of the hospital yesterday. His AGC was 1,264. But when they were getting ready to take his IV out, the nurse, Eve, told us his blood culture had grown something and they were calling Dr. Pizzo, the infectious disease expert.

Tears came to Jeff's eyes; I knew what he was thinking. The throat ached and I admit, fear knotted in my stomach. I told him not to worry and wiped his tears away. I said we would deal with whatever they were talking about. I had to really fight the tears from coming. I have to be strong for Jeff. At that time Scott May walked in the door. Thank you, Lord, for sending a friend. He sat with us and talked until the doctors came. They told us they felt it was nothing. Just a contaminate from the lab. Oh, how my heart leaped. Jeff was smiling a big smile. Oh, thank you Lord, I said in my heart. I said, "Jeff, did you say your prayers?"

"I sure did," he said. "Only me and God knows" and smiled a great big smile. Thank you, Lord! Sometimes, you feel you are going to be swallowed up with fear, hurt, and anxiety, but the Lord gives us strength. Oh, how I need His strength. We get so tired, very tired, and Jeff hurts so much. Pain from chemotherapy and now he is getting radiation every day. We are trusting in the Lord who has all the power to touch Jeff's body and restore his health. I pray that Jeff's body, each and every cell, will be cleansed from this cancer. Oh, God, we pray for a cure for this dreadful disease. So many young people we have seen here, suffering, and you say within yourself, "why, why."

But there are no answers. Someday, we will understand, but most of all when the Lord comes back to set things right in this world, there will be no more suffering. Praise the Lord!

We've learned to lean on Jesus. All day that song has come to my mind, learning to lean on Jesus. "Where could we go, but to the Lord?" ("Where could I go?" Hymn).

You know, how could Jack live in Houston with someone else and his son fighting cancer and his daughter has to live with relatives? God, I don't understand. There is just so much hurt, and I guess down deep anger for what he has done to our family. The Bible says, "Be angry but sin not," I guess I have enough love for Jack to overcome the hurt and anger because I really do pray for him. I guess what I really want is for him to want to come home and be a family, but greater than that, I pray for his relationship with God, and I pray that my concern for his soul and not to just satisfy my ego. But even if we didn't ever get back together, I do pray he will make things right with God. I don't even know if I could live with Jack anymore. O, Lord, what do you want me to do?

The Bible reminds me, "Be patient. Wait upon the Lord." In Him, we are trusting. We are looking with faith to the future and living each day on His strength and love.

When the tears and fears come, we just have to look to Jesus Christ, our Lord and Savior. He said he would be with us even to the end of the world.

And time and time again, when worry and fear tried to invade our thoughts. "Jesus said, 'I will come and heal him'" (Matthew 8:7).

That is our promise we are holding onto. Learning to lean on Jesus.

When Jeff had surgery (St. Mary's Hospital, Huntington, WV) and they came out and told us it was cancer, I passed out. But when they were putting me on the cot, I felt being lifted, my body lifted by caring hands, but now I know I was being spiritually lifted. The peace I felt. Thank you, Lord, for your loving kindness.

In God We trust.

✝

Sunday
February 3, 1985

Well, time is passing. Jeff went in the hospital, Thursday, for chemo. He really didn't get quite as sick this time, but it took three IVs to get him through the chemo. His veins have just been through it, and they just kept getting infiltrated. Jeff's getting really homesick, and sometimes, I know he would like to cry. But he always comes out of it. I wonder what Jeff really feels down deep inside. I think I can pretty well tell, but none of us know all of each other's inner thoughts. But I am so glad God does, and his Son is sitting on the right hand of God, interceding for us, and the Holy Spirit bears witness of this transaction. Praise the Lord for something I can feel!

Jeff has two more weeks of radiation and on February 19, he has all his reevaluation tests, bone scan, pelvic scans, chest scans, and his heart scan is on February 15. So, on February 20, we should be able to fly home for a couple of weeks. Oh, we pray for the outcome of the test to be negative and his heart scan to be okay. But, you know I really feel in my heart that the Lord has already touched Jeff, and this treatment working through the doctors is just a continuation of the healing process because I feel there is a reason for us being here, the people we have met, the doctors and nurses, and being away from home. I don't really understand, but we are trusting in the Lord, the author and finisher of our faith! Praise the Lord for the loving kindness, healing hand, his saving grace through his shed blood. Oh, thank the Lord. I feel so inadequate, so unworthy, and I do want to serve him to dissolve my will to totally be surrendered to the will of the Father.

And you know, I want for my children to follow the Lord, because He is leading us home, really home. Happiness, true happiness, no more suffering, no more tears, just everlasting eternal life with our Lord and Savior.

And again I have a feeling deep down inside that the Lord has something for Jeff to do and say. Someday we will understand and know. And you know Anita has been through so much. I know she has had marvelous family and friends with her but yet she is without her home and family. I think Anita has become a stronger Christian during this because she has also learned to lean on the Lord. It is hard to say, but I think that is where living your life and how you live it is so important. What words cannot be spoken, actions can speak even louder.

I've been able to read my Bible a lot through this, and that is one thing I never seemed able to find time to do before. Those precious words, so many. I think I will start recording some of them in the back of this book. Words of our Savior, words recorded through people inspired by the Holy Spirit to write, so very, very important through all the ages and ever still in the present time! Thank you, Lord, for your precious Word of God, the Bible.

"In God We Trust!"

✝

Thursday
February 7, 1985

Well, we are at the motel. We got back early today, about eleven-thirty. Jeff is tired.

We also found out today that Jeff's radiations treatment will not end until February 22, on Friday. His reevaluation tests will probably be on Monday, February 25. So, we're going to be even longer than we thought.

It's sort of hard to swallow, even having to stay five or six days longer. But it hit me this morning when I got up. Moses and the children of Israel were in the wilderness for forty years, and I don't know why but, I just thought well if it has to be, then we will be and just keep looking to the Lord. Yesterday, I felt so nervous and anxious; I was miserable inside. I try to hide it all so Jeff won't be upset. He has enough on his mind.

I really miss Anita and our home, but for whatever reason, we have to be here. We want to seek God's will and trust in Him. I was really feeling bad yesterday, sick headache. I felt that I was going to give in to worry and panic. But the Lord always comes, and I feel his precious presence, the comfort, the Holy Spirit. Such an appropriate name, the Comforter, because surely that is what the spirit of the Lord brings—comfort—along with that strength.

You know, sometimes, I hurt so badly especially after Jack calls. Like yesterday, he kept asking how I felt, and I think about saying, "What do you care, really care?" I hurt because I do need him and love him, and I need someone to hold me and tell me they love me, and you know I always thought Jack did love me. How could I have been so wrong? Then Jack tells me if we need him, just call. He could be here the next day. I don't know, I wish I could figure out what Jack really feels. I get so burdened down with it all. I just have to lean on Jesus and give Him our burdens. I say ours. I guess I mean mine, Jeff's and Anita's.

But even now, my heart is breaking for everything, but the Bible verse found in Romans 12:12 comes to my mind often, "Rejoice in hope, patient in tribulations, continuing instant in prayers."

We claim the promise and truths given to us in God's Holy Word. God cannot and will not lie, and there is no other God, and the One and only true God has all the power. He made the universe, our bodies, and fashioned by Him in His image.

We look not to a weak, sleeping God that does not hear or see. We look to the creator of our lives and the keeper of our very souls. That's power and victory, now and forever.

"*In God We Trust*"

✝

Monday
February 11, 1985, 4:15 p.m.

Well, we're in the hospital now, again. Jeff has a fever. This is his last fever period until March when he goes through the intense part of his treatment. Jeff has slept off and on all day. I think the nurses worry about him being depressed because he covers his head with his blanket and sleeps. But he always does this the first couple of days of his fever period. I really feel Jeff is handling all this better than I could. It's hard to explain. He very seldom complains. When he hurts really bad, he sometimes cries but never to the point of giving up. He laughs, talks, jokes, looks to the future with a quiet faith and determination. Maybe the word to use is assurance. He really has something inside; I can see it and feel it. One of the doctors came in today and she said, "It was a pleasure trip to come and see Jeff." Jeanette, the nurse, that was trying to decide if Jeff was depressed, she said about his handling all this, he's different. You know, I know how he is different. He has Jesus dwelling inside, that Holy Spirit, that Comforter.

Oh, praise the Lord for His mercy and loving kindness.

Thanks, be unto God! You know, I really feel Jeff has already been touched. He has God's Holy Seal on him and I'm not sure if I even comprehend what that means. But I know these human thoughts come and creep in, trying to take us over. But out Lord provides. He is ever with us, he said he would never leave us nor forsake us. Our Lord and Savior is with us. And the feeling that I had the morning of Jeff's surgery, I was so burdened to the point of collapse.

But when I came to myself, I experienced a deep feeling of peace, one I couldn't explain.

When I was lying there on that cot, I felt as though I was lying in the arms of Jesus. I knew I couldn't go on; so much had happened I couldn't go on. Jesus had to carry me. I know how weak I am. He is so strong. We're leaning on Him because my heart aches, and I sometimes think I can't go on. But my answer always comes.

Wait upon the Lord, have faith, be of good courage. *"My grace is sufficient for thee, for my strength is made perfect in weakness"* (2 Corinthians 12:9).

Oh, for the joy and peace He gives us. There is no peace and happiness to be found anywhere else.

Oh, God, I hurt inside for Jeff, his suffering, Jack's disobedience, my faults and failures. I should have been able to hold my marriage together, but I could not. Please forgive me, Lord. I need your help, I am worthless, and I beseech you for your help in our lives, healing of Jeff's body, Jack's relationship with thee, Anita, all of us. We need you. There is none other!

"In God We Trust"

✝

Saturday
February 16, 1985

Well, Jeff is feeling better. His fever is gone. His counts are up. We'll probably get out to the motel tomorrow. We can rest and relax a lot better out there.

Seems I'm getting nervous and anxious inside. I think it is when I get really physically tired. Jack just called. He seems to want talk a lot more now. I thought maybe he was wanting things different, but I don't think so. After we hung up, I went to the family room hospital phone and called Jack's number. A woman answered the phone, so I guess nothing has changed. He will go home to her. It hurts so bad. I should not have called. She just said hello, and I hung up. I just had to know. That is the first time I have even dialed that number since Jack went to Texas. I have to let go, don't I? But it is so hard, a lifetime, two children, a belief in marriage as sacred. How did all this happen? I can't even answer that. But so many things burden my heart and life right now. All I ever wanted and prayed for was a Christian home to raise my children in with love and God's love in it. I want my children to be healthy and serve the Lord. I tried to live as the Lord would want. But I have miserably failed. I couldn't even keep my husband. That I don't understand. I love him so much, and I guess I still do or it wouldn't hurt so much.

Dear Lord, what do you want me to do? I've prayed for Jack and still he is gone, and he has not professed a relationship with God. I guess he has the kind of life he wants. I wonder what he feels for me and if he really is happy. How could he be, his two children and Jeff sick, and all he can do is call on the telephone.

But Lord, I've come too far to turn back now, and I know you will take care of us. I believe Jeff will get well. I feel and believe in my heart that the Lord has plans for Jeff. I believe the Bible, God's word, and we will not despair!

I don't know how I can work around my marriage failure, but with the Lord's guidance and help, it will work out. Even though he is living with that woman, why do I feel that there is still hope? After all that has happened, how could it be? No other way, but through and by the Lord. I want to work for the Lord. I believe time is short. Souls are lost. We need to be about our Father's business. Jack has hurt me too much to describe with words. He has hurt the children, but I still pray for him that he will make things right with the Lord. I guess that is all that really matters.

"Lord, please help us, I fail sometimes and then in one of those times, I feel as though I'm sinking in a world of hurt. We are looking to our Lord, Praise His name forever!"

"In God We Trust!"

*****

Thursday
February 21, 1985

Boy, a week has almost passed, a good week. Although, Jeff didn't feel good for a couple days. We went to bed early Sunday night when we got out of the hospital. We were exhausted; I slept until one the next day. Jeff slept until about three. We don't get much sleep at the hospital. The last night that we were there, they brought Jim Nalty down from intensive care. He's about nineteen years old, in college, and wants to be a dentist. He has leukemia. He was still breathing with oxygen. He had been on a respirator, and he hiccupped all night. It just made me sick to see him suffer. I think of little Tisha, age four, who has leukemia; Danny, six months old, Rhabdo cancer; Raymond, age sixteen, leukemia; Domingo Allen, age twenty-two, leukemia; Alice, age sixteen, Rhabdo; Blaine, age sixteen, Ewing's; Mike Dokken, age nineteen, Ewing's; Johnny Toppings, age sixteen, Rhabdo; names and names. So much heartache and suffering. That's when you can look to Heaven and plead for Jesus Christ to come and stop this suffering but then you get the answer. *Just wait, my child, I know you are suffering, but there is a plan.* And now more than ever, I realize that God has not had the final say so yet, and He will, some-day, someday!

We just have to trust in Him and keep our faith!

There is so much to tell, and it's getting late. Mother called the other night and was telling us about grandpa getting sick, and she had to take him to the hospital. It was really bad; slick roads. Jeff started crying and said, "I don't want anything to happen to Pippie (my dad)," and with tears in his eyes, he said, "I wanna go to church!" Oh, thank you, Father. Since Jeff got home, he wanted his Bible. He put the oil cloth in it (I'll explain about that later), picked out what he said was his favorite Bible verse. *"I will never leave thee, nor forsake thee" (Hebrews 13:5).*

Then he said he wanted to go to the Bible book store and get some scripture cards. He also said he wanted to read the whole Bible. Oh, praise the Lord! Thanks, be unto God, our Father! I pray he will do just that.

Well, I'll write again soon, much more to write.

In God We Trust.

✝

Sunday
February 24, 1985

Well, it's finally here, our long-awaited trip home. Anita is here. We go to the hospital in the morning for Jeff's bone scan. Our plane leaves at 1:55 p.m. We've waited and thought it was so long, and now it's here. It will be good to relax at home for a few days. HOME—a word that we've thought about, how it's changed, but oh, Lord we're trusting in thee. Last week while Jeff was in the hospital (this is the much more I wanted to write), he started crying, he was worried about Pippie driving to Huntington to take Grandpa to the hospital on icy roads. He said, "I don't want anything to happen to Grandpa. I wanna go home; I wanna go to church." My heart really bursts with happiness, sadness, joy, and sorrow, all at the same time. Oh Lord, I don't understand so much hurt and suffering in our lives in the last year and a half. But I feel a plan; God's plan is being worked out. I just pray we will do God's will. We don't know the future; it's in God's hands and that is our security, safe in the arms of Jesus. He sits at God's right hand. He hears our prayers! You know, I was reading an article in a book. It said when God says "yes," we gratefully say thank you. When he says "no," we accept it. But when God says "wait," we have a really hard time, and that's true. I feel we sometimes have to wait for God's plan to be worked out. I believe God has touched Jeff, and healing can be a process, during which time, His will is carried out. We just have to look to the all-wise Heavenly Father. I know and believe He knows our cries and feels our heartaches. God will answer our prayers. I feel deep inside God has work for Jeff to do. Life is short, souls are lost, and we must be about our Father's business. I do so little and am so unworthy, but I know He loves me, and I ask His forgiveness and thank Him and praise His name forever.

"In God We Trust!"

✝

Wednesday
March 13, 1985

I have not written for two weeks. We went home and were so busy I didn't write. When we got off the plane, we found out my grandfather had died. We went to the funeral on Wednesday, February 27. He was eighty-seven years old, Floyd Wysong, my mother's father. Jeff also went to the funeral. He wanted to go. We had a lot of company and I worked six days. I never get to bed before one or two o'clock any night. Sunday night before we came back, I was up until 4:00 a.m. I guess I had a lot to do, and I couldn't get settled down. We flew up here and to the Colonial Manor. We went to the mall, and then Jeff ate New York Strip at Manny's at the Colonial Manor. Ben Sebastian and his family came up for a little while.

  We came to the hospital yesterday. They put Jeff's central line in his neck. I thought I was going to be sick. They numbed his neck and slit it and inserted a tube which he will receive intravenous feeding and antibiotics through. Jeff just laid there. I don't know how he does it, facing all the things, but I guess I do know. His faith in our Lord, Jesus Christ sustains him. This morning he had total body radiation. I watched him on the screen. He had to sit on a chair, twenty minutes on each side. My heart broke for him, watching him. He was sleepy from the medication they gave him, and his head hung down from nodding. He got so uncomfortable, leg cramps and every once in a while, he would cry out and moan. You could see the pain in his face. Oh, my God it hurts so much! I thought my heart would break into pieces. I prayed, "Dear Heavenly Father, please sustain him through this," and he made it. Jeff has a lot of fortitude. I know where that comes from, Praise the Lord. The Bible says Jesus' own words in Matthew 7:7, "Ask and it shall be given to you." Matthew 21:22 also says "and all things, whatsoever ye shall ask in prayer, believing, ye shall receive." Ask and ye shall receive.

I believe in my heart the Heavenly Father has heard not only my prayers but many on Jeff's behalf. Even when it gets so bad and I hurt beyond words of description, I feel in my heart, Jesus says just wait, have faith, you will see, and somehow, I see and feel a time when Jeff will declare unto the world the Lord's salvation and soon coming King. I also believe time is short, and there is much labor to be done.

Every time we come here to this hospital, we find out more have relapsed and some have died. They tell me Blaine Prince died. Just two or three months ago, I saw him, so handsome, and I talked with his mom. It hurts so deeply and can be very disturbing. But we are looking to the One who can beat all odds. They tell us Ewing's Sarcoma has a 40 percent cure rate. The doctors, especially, Dr. Miser, knows that God is the final answer. Even if there were no percentage of cure rate, it takes only for our Lord to say the word; healing will come through and by our Lord and Savior. I know He feels our heartache and pain. He, himself, suffered so much for us and how He prayed. My heart cries out and He sustains us. I need His strength. Sometimes, especially now during this intensive, I feel I'm on the verge of collapse, physically, mentally, and emotionally. But I get the same answer when I look to the Heavenly Father and His Son crucified and resurrected, and now alive forever more.

"I can do all things through Christ which strengthens me" (Philippians 4:13).

Praise the Lord forever! Oh, how I love Jesus!

"In God We Trust!"

＋

Friday
March 22, 1985

Well, today is Friday. We've been here ten days now. Jeff has had all his treatments now. Six months of treatment, his intensive consisting of two days total body radiation, two days chemo, 1,200 mg cytokine, 35 mg Adriamycin, 2 mg Vincristine. His day of rest was last Sunday. Then on Monday, he got his bone marrow back. I haven't written since last Wednesday. Seems I just couldn't write, maybe just too much burden right now. When Jeff was going through total body radiation and chemo, I just couldn't talk about it even. It hurt so much to see Jeff suffer, but he never really seems bitter. Although he did say he thought about telling his dad what he thought about things. He started crying and said he has four weeks of vacation and sick leave, and he should be here and stay longer than four or five days if he really cared. I told him not to worry about it, and he said, "What am I supposed to do? Mom, I have cancer. I don't expect any special treatment, but he should be here." What can I say? I just don't know how to deal with Jack anymore.

Anyway, the bone marrow reinfusion was something he should have been here for. The doctors, Dr. Miser, Dr. Stice, and another doctor and Jeff's nurse, Jeanette and I were present. We all had to wear mask and surgical hats in case one of the bone marrow boxes cracked during thawing. They brought a steel box container in which Jeff's bone marrow had been stored since December 21, 1984, in a dry ice solution. When you open the box, steam comes out. They took one bag out at a time and thawed it in a hot sterile solution.

Then Dr. Stice hung it on Jeff's IV pole and ran it through his IV. It was a very moving experience. I thank God for the marvelous medical technology and doctors. God has allowed man so much knowledge and medicine to treat cancer. But I hope and pray for a cure for this disease. Praise God, let them find a cure for all these children. After he got the reinfusion, he vomited and started chilling and shaking. They gave him Thorazine for vomiting and Demerol for chills. He went to sleep and slept for about four hours. The smell was pretty bad in the room. I got a little nauseous, too. Jeff kept cinnamon certs in his mouth, so he said it wasn't that bad. So, after that, he felt pretty good except for nausea. We played chess, trivial pursuit every night, and yesterday, we went to the fourteenth floor and he pushed his IV pole around the pool table and played a game of pool.

Well, last night he got a fever of 38.5 C (101.3F). About eleven-thirty we went downstairs and got a chest X-ray, and they started him on antibiotics. So now we wait. I hope and pray his throat and nose don't get really sore.

Ben Sebastian and his mom just came to visit. They are really good friends and Christian people. So now we wait and hope and pray for his counts to come up. His nose and throat and tongue are bothering him pretty much.

I just pray for strength right now. I feel in my heart the Lord is watching over Jeff. The Bible speaks of ministering angels, and I believe that Spirit or whatever you might call it is ever present at Jeff's bedside.

Well, I'm going downstairs to get Ben a gift. He brought Jeff a little teddy bear that says God loves you. May God bless and heal Ben too. Thank you, Lord, for all your marvelous grace and promises. "Wait on the Lord, be of good courage" (Psalm 27:14). That's what we're doing.

"In God We Trust"

✝

Sunday
March 24, 1985

It's 9:30 p.m. Jeff had a pretty tough night. His nose bled and ran down the back of his throat, and he vomited. His hemoglobin dropped to 6.6, and his platelet count to 7,000. The cut off for transfusion is 8.5 and platelet 20,000. He got platelets twice yesterday and two units of blood.

Wednesday
March 27, 1985

Well, it's Wednesday and I haven't been able to write because Jeff has been pretty sick. But Praise the Lord, He is here with us! Jeff is suffering; he has sores all over his tongue and throat and can barely swallow. He's going to get two units of blood today. His fever went up to 39.1 C. They tried ice packs, and then they put him on a cooling blanket Monday night. It is very uncomfortable and very cold. His fever did come down to 37.9 this morning, but it is now 38.4 C. They say it will fluctuate. But praise the Lord, his WBC is 100 today. It has been less than 100 for two days now. Tomorrow, we pray we will see more of a rise in his WBC. It has been hard, but I know and thank God for His marvelous presence we have felt. Our natural eyes cannot see Jesus standing, watching over Jeff's bedside, His Spirit touching every fiber, muscle, bone, cell, in Jeff's body. Oh, the power of God and marvelous love that sent His son to the cross to die for us. I think through all of this, it has made me more aware of God's love, and how it must have grieved his heart beyond description. Oh, what love and Jesus's mother as she stood at the foot of the cross. Someday, just think of it, we will be able to live in the very presence of the Almighty God and kneel at Jesus's feet and talk with Mary and all those saints of yesterday. What joy fills our heart. There is so much more than just life, which is so short and full of suffering. Oh, how I love Jesus, for His sacrifice and shed blood, promises, touching, healing Jeff's body. Oh, I could write until my life is over and never thank Him enough. My wonderful daughter, Anita, a loving, forgiving heart, which only God's love can give. I still pray for Jack and love him to want God's love to fill his life also.

"In God We Trust"

✝

Well, days and nights have passed since I have written, many sleepless and tiring nights. Jeff has been pretty sick with fever, low platelets causing nose bleed, nausea, vomiting blood, and low hemoglobin. He has awakened frequently during the night, and most of the time, there has been nurses and doctors coming in and out. It has been pretty bad, and Jeff has suffered, sore mouth and throat. But I know in my heart, we have much to be thankful for, and I do, from my very being, give all glory and praise to the Heavenly Father. There are so many things; his bone marrow started working on the eighth day, his tongue healed up almost overnight, and he did get the new branch chain amino acids which they think really help during this intensive. Dr. Miser who is over the Ewing's protocol comes by, and he once told Jeff that the Lord was really helping him. He said last Thursday Jeff was doing good but unfortunately had to go on Amphoterious, an anti-fungal agent which does knock the fever. He was on ceftazidine and Flagyl, anti-bacterial antibiotics for seven days. After that, you have to go to ampho.

The first dose, Friday sent his temperature soaring to 40.7 degrees Celsius (105 F). He had to stay on the cooling blanket until Saturday. Each ampho dose makes your temperature go up, but it does come back down. His WBC Saturday and Sunday were 400, and today it was 600 with 28 polys which is equal to 168 AGC. It has to be over five hundred before we can come off the antibiotics. They are tapering his morphine to 6 mg over two hours instead of 10 mg. They will also have to taper him off the TPN. He still cannot eat. He's been on TPN three weeks Wednesday and hasn't eaten anything in over a week. But he did eat a popsicle and two jelly beans yesterday. Oh, I pray to our Heavenly Father, please heal his body and let him take nourishment and bring his counts up. Dr. Miser said pray the counts up, and I said I have been and that we never stop praying. Oh, so many have been and are praying. Thank you, Lord, for our Christian friends and family that know the worth of prayers. Our revival is starting at church this week. I pray God's family will be uplifted and revived and many souls born into Gods family.

I pray for my daughter, Anita. She is young, and I ask the Heavenly Father to watch over her and lead, guide and direct her life and all her decisions, and that she is receptive to God's will. You know I'm thinking about our lives, returning home and to a "normal" life but, somehow, I know it will not be like before, maybe normal but not the same. We will need God's strength in the days ahead as we try to recover from the trauma of such an illness, and I pray for Jeff. Oh, God, in Jesus's name I pray for him. To give him strength mentally, physically, and emotionally to return to a "normal" life, back to school, old friends, but again I feel like it will not be the same. God's plan is in the working here. I can feel it, sense it. I know not exactly the plan, but I am trusting in the Lord, God Almighty, Jeff, as we all are, is in His hands and I feel much that God has a work for Jeff to do. We can only look to Him as we cannot see the future. I pray with all my heart for Jeff's future that he will look to the Lord for strength and guidance and ever follow where he leads. I know "quiet" Jeff loves the Lord and his faith is anchored there.

"In God We Trust"

✝

Tuesday
April 2, 1985

Well, it's 12:30 p.m., Jeff is getting his Ampho. They gave him morphine and then Benadryl, so he is sleeping. His WBC is 700 today. His platelet count dropped to 2,000 this morning, very low, but he got an O positive transfusion this a.m., so I hope it really helps him stay up there. He also got potassium. His potassium was 2.9. It's a recovery process now, waiting on the counts to come up.

Jack and all his family went home Saturday. When Jack was leaving, he was crying after he told Jeff bye, and I met him in the hallway. He said, "Well Linda, I'll see you." I said okay, that's it and he left. I thought my heart would break. I'm not exactly sure why. It did hurt me that he was crying, but it all hurts me; what could have been.

But while Jack was here, I guess I really saw him for the way he is, a womanizer, a woman chaser, a liar, deceitful, and self-centered. He sat out front and guess who he made friends with. About three women, who I guess are the type he likes. Those that drink and carry on with filth, a dirty mouth. He left one evening, last Thursday, about seven and was gone for about two hours or more. He did not tell me or Jeff where he was going. I went out front to the bathroom and Pat Norfors said, "Your ex must be having one hell of a time with those ladies he went out with," and I said, "I don't even know where he is. He didn't even tell us he was leaving." She couldn't believe it. But the Friday before, he said he was going to a friend's house to spend the night. He left no number he could be reached at. Another night, Pat told me, that last Friday night they called him from the Colonial Manor Motel, wanting him to come over and have some drinks, Jackie, Carol, and Pat. He didn't go, but I was told Carol came back here, drunk, and half raped him. Sickening, sickening, even in a hospital under these circumstances, people can't control Satan's evilness. Oh, God help. I do pray for those people, but it hurts; always behind my back he does these things. How long had these things been going on? I loved him, and I trusted him, and he betrayed me, lied, and cheated. Well, he doesn't have to answer to me, but he will have to answer to the Lord God Almighty. I pray for his soul. Jack turn around before it's too late. These women will have to answer too, all of them.

He comes up here and is here a few days and tries to tell everyone to hang in there; he calls and says the same thing. He doesn't know what it means to hang in there; he couldn't even hang in a marriage and fulfill his vows and he has the nerve! Well, I deal and pray about these feelings. We are instructed to love and pray for our enemies. I guess Jack would be my enemy. He sought to use me and take advantage and used my love and trust to cover his lies and deceitfulness. I don't understand how anyone can do that, but it sure happens very often these days. No one seems to really care, and they take their marriage vows even less seriously.

O, God, if I wronged by divorcing Jack, please forgive me. It seemed I have no choice, and I felt I had done everything I could do, and it was just in your hands. I need guidance, Lord, to say and do the things that would be pleasing unto thee. Maybe Jack being here at this hospital helped to open my eyes. I didn't like very much what I saw.

"In God We Trust"

✝

Well, it's 4:45 p.m. Scott May came over and spent the day with us and brought us breakfast. Scott has been a true friend. He's called us and visited us, always asking if we needed anything. He's a good boy from down home that's working up here.

Jeff is really frustrated. His counts keep going up and down. He wants out of here. He's done really good all through this, but I guess everyone has a breaking point. It's bad enough to deal with cancer and this treatment, but Jeff is dealing with feelings of rejection from Jack. Oh, I know how that hurts! Jeff has cried and cried because he says Jack doesn't love him. He cried for his daddy and wants him to come home and come back up here. I told him that Jack left me and that he doesn't love me but that he loves them (Anita and Jeff) but Jeff said, "No, Mom, he left all of us, and he doesn't love any of us." What do you say when the fact is he did leave all of us, not just going to Houston, long before then, even when he was still living at home. Oh, what a foolish thing to do, to leave a loving family. O God, help me not to build hatred in my heart. I do love Jack, and I don't want him to be lost, but I can't judge, only God can do that. But I know Jeff is hurting very much for the love of his father. But, Lord, what can I do? I can't make him come home, and if I have to make him or if because of Jeff's illness, what good would it do? Only cause more hurt for the kids and me. Jack caused a lot of hurt even when he was home because he wasn't part of us as a family. I know the Bible says a righteous partner will influence the other. Why couldn't I influence

Jack? He let the world influence him above his family and friends. O, Lord what will the future hold? Again, I must say, we just have to lean on Jesus. That is our hope and anchor.

I pray for Jeff; give him strength, we're still here in the fourteenth floor waiting room. Oh, please God help us. I feel so tired and weak. Jeff's spirits are down. We need to feel God's uplifting.

"In God We Trust"

†

Tuesday
April 9, 1985

Well, it's 7:30 a.m. I just got up and got dressed. We slept really good last night. Jeff's toes hurt and he took a codeine tablet and it helped.

Well, there is so much to write about Sunday (Easter Sunday). I guess I'll start at the beginning. I got up and went to the protestant church service on the fourteenth floor at 10:00 a.m.

They had communion. I couldn't let an Easter Sunday go by without going to church and thanking my Savior. There were about twenty people there. We each introduced ourselves there were people from all over the country there; Wisconsin, New York, Maine, and West Virginia. Jeanette, the nurse, said she would take care of Jeff while I was gone. Then after church, Anita called and told us that Jeff Clay was being baptized today (Easter Sunday).

We then had a dinner, ham, egg, etc. The parents that were out-patient brought food, and we divided the cost $16 each. It was nice; families away from home sharing Easter Sunday and sufferings of our children. Pat and Bill Norfors' son Danny, who is now ten months old, has Rhabdo (a muscle cancer) and it has spread to his lungs. The doctors told her she could just take him home and try phase 1 treatment, which is purely experimental. They have decided to try the experimental. The dinner was kind of sad. I held Danny for a while, and he just smiled at Jeff and me. Jeff has really been upset about Danny. We were out front practically all evening. Then about seven, we went up to the fourteenth floor to see the city lights at night. Jeff said, "It's beautiful, ain't it, Mom?" as far as you can see, lights. Then we went to the chapel and sat awhile and had a silent prayer. That has sort of become a habit. It's so peaceful to go there. Last night we went (Monday), Jeff said he loved to go there, that he just could sleep all night there. My heart leaps with joy and feels burdened at the same time. I felt I just want to come and say "Thank you Lord" for His saving grace, His healing power, His calming spirit in the midst of trial and suffering, His marvelous promises and love. I could go on forever and never praise Him adequately. Last night, Jeff started to cry, while we were in the chapel. He said just everything, wanted to go home, he wanted Anita. He has been through so much.

Sunday night we came back downstairs, and Anita called after church and told us some very good news. The revival did not close. Basil Vickers got saved! Praise the Lord! I fixed a prayer list I carry with me in my pocketbook, and that makes three people I can place a check beside of in the last year that has gotten saved. I have prayed for them every day. Praise the Lord forever more. He does answer prayers. Jeff's illness is on the prayer list also. I placed a check some time ago. I feel in my heart and thank God; he has touched and healed Jeff from this terrible disease. You know these thoughts of doubt try to creep in, especially here you see a relapse almost every day or hear of someone dying. But dear Heavenly Father, we look unto thee, You said to ask, and we have asked, and I feel you have heard and answered. I don't know why all this happened, but there is a reason, even when things have looked bad, and Jeff has been so sick. I can see victory and God's plan. We'll understand someday. We travel through this life either in despair or faith and hope. God gave us a choice. He sent His son to make a way. I choose God, His son crucified and resurrected, sitting on the right hand of God, interceding for us. Oh, just think, what power we have in our hearts, in our very possession. He's listening for us to cry out to Him. I'm so weak and tired but He is so strong! We don't deserve His love and death for us, but He answers our prayers because He loves us. He is wanting to hear from us.

"O, God, ever remind us to seek the wisdom and power in Christ Jesus's name. O Lord, forgive my faults, my weakness, and my unworthiness. I give myself to thee. Help us to know thy will. Thank you Lord!"

Also, Scott May went to church Sunday night, for the first time in three years.

"In God We Trust"

✝

Monday
April 15, 1985

Today is Jeff's birthday. He is fifteen years old. So much has happened already in his young life. But praise the Lord, we are trusting in Him. Our future, Jeff's, Anita's, and mine, we lay in His hands. My prayers for my children are that they will always live for the Lord, do His will and I know and believe that everything will be okay. God is all powerful; we have nothing to fear. He will take care of us. He said he would hear us and answer. He knows our very inner thoughts.

We have talked to everyone; Anita, Wanda and family, Mother, Daddy, Fay, Eric, Tish, Mamaw Salmons, and Jack. I really feel I should just let Jack talk to the kids. If he doesn't want his home, then it's about time I let go. I guess these feelings are just pent-up hurt feelings. I want to do what is right according to God's will. I can pray for Jack. I don't hate him, but I don't think I have to hold on to his presence or talking to him. I don't love anyone else. Roger is a friend, but I don't feel anything for him or anyone. If the Lord wants me to have a mate, I'll just have to pray about it. Would it be wrong? I don't think so, really, under the circumstances, but I would really have to search my heart and pray.

Well, we got out of the hospital last Wednesday, April 11. We arrived here at the motel about 4:30 p.m. The family, Anita, Mother, Daddy, Wanda, David, and Davey arrived then, too. So, we had some good visiting. We went to the National Zoo on the subway and went fishing on the Potomac River. Jeff really enjoyed that. They all went home Saturday about noon. We really miss them. But hopefully, we will get to come home by the end of the week. They have to make sure his potassium and platelets are okay. Jeff has done really good and I know we have so much to be thankful for. I want to list some, for in time to come; we might forget just what to Lord has done. To begin with, I feel He worked it out for us to come here. It has been tough, but I feel it was in God's plan. The treatment has really been rough. He developed a fiche, a tear in his rectum which really hurt him bad one week when he had a fever. The nurses and doctors all said it would really be bad during intensive but praise the Lord, it healed, and it did not bother him at all during the intensive. He gained a little muscle. He was on TPN (intravenous feeding) for four weeks. There is a new TPN (branch chain amino acids—40 percent) they randomize. I prayed he would get the new if it would help. He got the new. I prayed his bottom would heal and it did, and his counts started working on the eighth day. He walked into the hospital, and he walked out. *Praise the Lord!* He's eating now. He has only had to get platelets one time since checking out of the hospital. During his TBI and chemo, he was playing chess and Trivial Pursuit or something every evening. The nurse said Jeff was different, had an inner strength. Jeff trusted in the Lord, prayed to Him. That is his inner strength.

O, Lord we have so much to be thankful for. We're trusting in thee to get home soon. We miss Anita so much. Please be with her, dear Lord. Thank you, Lord!

In God We trust.

Sunday
May 19, 1985

Well, it's Sunday morning. I'm sitting on the porch and everyone around us is pulling out to go to church. We've been home one month yesterday. Jeff has not felt very well. I've been so busy working. I really feel I need to be home, but if I don't go to work, I don't get paid. My pay check ran out because I am out of sick leave.

Jeff has lost ten more pounds. He couldn't eat for about two weeks. His back hurts him when he lies on his right side or sits up. Just last night, he had a fever. Oh, God, it's like living in the shadow of a big wall just ready to fall anytime. The doubts move in, fear, and oh, how it hurts to see Jeff suffer. But I still believe in God's power and promises. Hope, that's all we have. Only one place to look to, that is our Heavenly Father. Am I weak? Am I doubting God, because I hurt, worry, and live with that fear of Jeff's cancer coming back? His back hurting gnaws at me constantly, the fever last night. But all I can say is that we're still trusting in the Lord. Please give me strength, Lord. Sometimes I think I'm going to collapse.

I worry about Anita, she's young, so much influences. We need to get back in church, and I pray Jeff will be able to attend Bible school. He wants to so much. I guess, Lord, sometimes I have so many feelings. Sometimes it's ecstatic joy and then deep despair, sometimes love, forgiveness, and sometimes hurt and deep anger. But these feelings, Lord, I feel love and reverence for a mighty God who sent his only begotten son to die for us, and I believe in the old rugged cross and what it did for us through Jesus Christ our Savior.

Who do we have to fear? God is all-powerful. Child of God, we will *not* lose.

In God We trust. We fly to Maryland Wednesday for test.

"In God We Trust"

✝

Thursday
May 30, 1985

Well, we're sitting here in the waiting area of NIH, waiting for the shuttle to come and go to the airport to go home. Jeff has had all of his tests, and praise the Lord, they were all good. They found he had a urinary infection and have put him on an antibiotic. That is what has been causing the fever. Oh, God, thank you for your loving kindness and healing power. Just before we came up here, I was reading Psalms, and there is a verse in Psalm 56 that reads, "When I am afraid, I will put my trust in Thee" (v. 3). That verse has been in my mind and heart ever since. It has sustained me. Praise the Lord! I admit I was afraid and hurt so much for Jeff. Jeff is so quiet, but somehow, I feel he has so much faith inside, a quiet faith. The Lord sustains him, too. We're just leaning on Jesus and trusting in the almighty God our Father for the future.

I dreaded coming in a way. I wanted to find out the cause of Jeff's fever, but I dreaded going to the sixth floor and finding out who has died—Jim Nulty (leukemia), Stephanie Gormby (Atkinson cancer), Bobby Travers (leukemia), Danny Norfors (rhabdo); Dawn, George's daughter, died just yesterday. Oh, Heavenly Father, please be with those families. We also learned Albert (leukemia) has relapsed, and Steven Cloreson, (Ewing's), had relapsed. There is so much dying and suffering around us. We just have to look to our Heavenly Father for strength. It hurts so much, all these children and their suffering. Well, we have to come back the last week in June for tests. We're going home, thankful and trusting in God for the future tests. God be with us is my prayer. I called Anita. She was so happy. Bless my children, Lord, in thy love and may we all live for thee and do thy blessed will.

"In God We Trust."

✝

August 7, 1985

Time flies. Life goes on. I can't believe I haven't written since May. We came back from Maryland, and Jeff started recuperating. There's so much to write. Praise the Lord! Jeff felt so bad from the treatment and urinary infection. He wanted to go to vacation bible school. I prayed for him to recover and feel like attending. Praise the Lord, he not only recovered, he attended every night, and Anita and Jeff made bust of Jesus. They are beautiful! Well, we had the Bible school wiener roast at our pastor's house, and we all went.

Then my mother and dad, Wanda, David, Davy and Lisa, and all of us plus Phil headed to go to the beach (Long Beach, North Carolina). Jeff's feet at the time were hurting him real bad (toes mostly). Well, we went. I drove all the way. But it was a good week. Jeff's feet quit hurting him, and he stopped taking codeine that week. Our pastor and other members of our church were there also, and we visited them some and hunted for sea shells. Well, we came back and was home five days (July 4) week, and then we left on Sunday, Anita, too for Maryland. We were there all week. Jeff has a bone marrow scan, pelvic and chest X-rays. Everything was okay, urine culture also. Praise the Lord! We don't have to go back until September 29 for a couple days. He will get all his scans then. That will be his five to six months out from treatment checkup. They say if you go five months and not relapse it is a good sign. But my, no, I'll say our signs, have been from God. A feeling from the heart, many prayers, an oil cloth, a leaf in a tree, December tests, and most important, Jeff's witness. Oh, thank you Lord for everything. We're trusting in the One who holds the future. When I look to September and October and remember the past, I admit it scares me, but I must remember Psalm 56:3. Oh, Lord, give us strength and courage to face each day. Well, we got home from Maryland, Friday, July 12 at 5:00 p.m. At 12:30 a.m., we were on our way to the beach again with Roger and his family.

I kept thinking, I can't believe I'm doing this, but we did, and we had a good week. On the way down, my car broke down just outside of Charlotte, North Carolina. After putting oil in it three times, we finally parked it and I called AAA and had it towed in. Roger's daughter Tammy's boyfriend, Ric, called his dad who lives in Charlotte, and he tried to borrow his friend's car for us, and it blew up, so he ended up taking us on to the beach. We had one car all week for nine people. We went in two shifts when we went out to eat or something. But mostly, Roger and I sat on the porch and drank our coffee and talked. We walked on the beach one night alone, and we found a gigantic seashell. I cooked breakfast every morning, grilled some. It was a good week for Jeff; he got plenty of exercise walking, trying to keep up with Dale. Anita, Phil, Tammy, and Ric went out some. David was with Roger and me mostly. I have a lot of confused feelings right now. Feelings for Roger, love for Jack, I don't know if I will ever get them sorted out or if Roger and I could have a relationship. Well, I had to leave my car in Charlotte, North Carolina. It wasn't fixed, no parts. So, we came back in Roger's car and Ric's car, he bought from his dad while we were down there.

I guess if you want to look on the bright side of things, if I hadn't gone, my warranty on my car probably would have run out before my car broke down. It broke down July 13; my warranty ran out July 25. Also, Jeff quit taking medication (Elavil) while we were down there. He only takes Tylenol now when he needs something. Roger spent the next week home with his mom and dad. His mom had her eye removed. She can hardly see out of the other. They are sweet people. He came up about three nights. I went to his mom and dad's with him. Oh, I just don't know what I feel. I ask the Lord for guidance.

So, we've finally been home for a while, resting, sleeping, cooking, and band practice started, all the normal things. Thank you,

Lord. All the normal things. It's raining now, and I'm sitting on the front porch. Thank you, Lord, for everything! Anita and Phil are in the house; Jeff and Eric are over at Eric's house. It's nice to be able to sit on the porch. I love to do that and look up at the sky and talk to God and thank Him and ask Him for help, strength, and guidance.

So normal life had resumed. It has been hard for Jeff. He feels so inadequate. He felt that a lot when Dale found him a girlfriend at the beach, and he didn't. Jeff looks like he has been through something recently but I believe someday Jeff will be and look healthy and strong according to God's will. So, I pray for Jeff to have patience, wait on the Lord. It will be better. Maybe he can't do some of the things he used to do (football etc.). But, the Lord may have other plans. Let us look to Him with faith and follow His will. Give Jeff the strength, courage, and boldness for thee, Lord, is my prayer. That prayer should and is for all of us, let us live for the Lord. Anita and Phil seem to really care for each other. Direct and guide them dear Lord, that they may follow according to your will and make the right decisions.

Jeff and Anita do not realize it but I see so much hurt in them sometimes, I could and do cry. It breaks my heart; I just do not understand how Jack could have ever done all those things and instead of trying to work things out and just leave. Help me to forgive him, dear Lord. I do pray for him. The Lord knows my heart, we can't hide anything.

Well, I did finally get my car back. David, Anita, and Phil, and I went and got it the next Wednesday after we got home (July 24).

I want to explain about the signs, feelings in depth the next time I write. You know we never know exactly how the Lord might answer our prayers or even send someone or something into our lives, but praise the Lord, we can say God does hear and answer prayers! I ask the Lord what I can do to thank Him and be a witness to glorify his name.

In God We Trust.

✝

September 15, 1985

Well another month or so has gone by. Boy, a busy time. School started, band, football, all the normal things. Praise the Lord. Thank you, Lord.

I get so tired physically and mentally, but yet I feel so good, it's hard to explain; it is the spirit dwelling inside. It has to be, it is. There's nothing in this world that gives one that feeling of peace, sweet assurance. It was promised by Jesus Christ Himself at his ascension. The Comforter would come when He went away, to comfort, guide, and lead, until Jesus returns for us. Oh, what a promise! What power! It seems sometimes I can almost see it, I feel, I sense, but I can't see it with a natural eye. I can see the effect of it. I can see where it has been, praise the Lord, but someday our eyes will be opened to behold all the glory and we can bow at His feet and say glory, glory, to the Son of God!

There's so much to tell and write. We have been pretty busy with school and everything. I was concerned that Jeff would have a hard time sitting at school every day but you know, he loves it and says it doesn't bother him. I ask the Lord to strengthen him and Jeff has gone to school every day and football practice every evening except one day. He can't play football. But he is helping manage the team. The first time I took him up there, he took his football pants from last year and I let him out of the car and watched him walk down the field to the coaches and players. I thought my heart would break and tears still come to my eyes when it comes to remembrance because I know how bad he wanted and wants to play. But then those tears turned to joy because I thought, well, if all he can do is carry the football to the boys and carry equipment and water, then praise the Lord! That's what he will do. The Lord maybe has other plans, maybe someday he will play, but maybe not, God's will be done, but I believe that according to God's will, it will be best for Jeff. I believe in God's promises. He will take care of us. Please, Lord, let us seek your will and wisdom.

We go back to NIH, September 29, for Jeff's checkup. He will get all of his scans and counts checked. I know what some people think that he won't be all right, but the Lord has all the power, even above the doctors! It's to Him we look and pray, and I feel in my heart God has already answered our prayers concerning Jeff's healing. You know, I said, and the Bible bears it out; St. John 3:8, the Spirit is as the wind, we can't see it, we hear it. We see the effects of it, but we "cannot tell whence it cometh and whether it goeth," there has been many effects of the Spirit over the last year. I want to write it down, maybe someday, somehow, to spread it far and wide, God hears and answers prayers. He sustains; He never leaves you (Hebrews 13:5). No matter what, Praise the Lord!

First, I want to start way back during the week Jeff had surgery and was in St. Mary's Hospital. The morning he had surgery, we were in the inner waiting room, Jack, Mickey, me, and sometimes Wanda or some other family member. Everyone else was in the outer waiting room. I was in such a state. I really don't know how to explain to anyone how I felt. It was like being in my body but feelings so deep I was also removed from that body. But I remember, a lady who was there with a friend having surgery. She talked continually, mostly about the Lord. I was so sick and deep in prayers and thought for Jeff I couldn't even talk much to her.

Well after about three hours, Dr. Smith came out and got us and said he removed the tumor, and that it was malignant, Ewing's Sarcoma. He also said the survival rate was not very good, and it was the worst kind to have. He said we needed to take him to the National Cancer Institute in Washington DC. Well, I got sick and passed out and I've already written what happened after that, but the story with the lady in the waiting room didn't end there! On the night before we left for DC, NIH, (Wednesday night), everyone had left the hospital. Jack was still there. I was out in the waiting room by myself. The elevator door opened, and this lady stepped out. She said, "You're who I'm hunting for," and I said, "I know you, don't I?"

She said, "I just came from church and we had a special prayer for your son, and the Lord told me to come and bring this oil cloth." She said the Lord is going to do something for him. I told her I had been thinking about anointing of oil. I had read a story in the Guidepost Magazine about it and I thought there was scripture on it, but no one around here that I know practices it. But sure enough (read James 5:14), this lady said their church practices this, and I ask her to come on back and see Jeff. She did and gave him the oil cloth and told him to wear it. We walked back to the elevator, and I told her, we might be of different denomination (I think her church is Pentecostal) on 4th Avenue, Huntington, West Virginia, but we were sisters in Christ and are serving the same Lord. She agreed and then she said, "We'll see each other again someday and surely we will, if not here, in the world to come!" She said, "If you were thinking about the anointing oil and the Lord told me to come, two hearts agree, then it had to be from the Lord."

Well, I pinned the oil cloth to Jeff's shirt, and he wore it all the time, only taking it off for X-rays, scans, etc. It is now pinned in his Bible. The tests he had in December, bone, biopsy, bone marrow, were all negative. I believe the answer, the healing, came straight from Heaven, from Almighty God. Praise the Lord. He sent this lady, a message of hope and promise. A strength through all of this, and I don't even know her name. What if she had waited one more day? We would have been gone to DC. The Lord sent her to the right place at the right time. It had to come from the Lord. Praise His name forever! What can I do to glorify His name? I feel Him leading, exactly where and what I don't know, but I will seek prayers, not just for me but to lead, guide, and direct my children. We need to be a witness for our Lord and Savior Jesus Christ!

Next, I want to write about the leaf on the tree at my mother and dad's house. There are many instances much more to write. We look to God for the results of September testing. I remember Psalm 56:3.

Thank you, Lord!

Praise the Lord.

"In God We Trust"

✝

Tuesday
October 8, 1985

Well, it's been a year. A year ago, today, Jeff entered the hospital for possible football injury. A year has passed, a very frightening, hurtful year of suffering! But the Lord has brought us through! Praise his name forever. I look where he brought us from and where we could have been.

This morning, Jeff wanted to go squirrel hunting with Davy. He didn't have anyone to go with, and Davy got off work today. I thought, a year ago today, Praise the Lord, he can walk a hill and go squirrel hunting. I let him go! Oh, thank you Lord. I can say thank you a hundred times a day, and it would not be enough. Well, we went to NIH on September 29, Sunday, and on Monday starting at 7:00 a.m., Jeff had IVP, cauterization, Voiding Cystogram, pelvic and chest X-ray, pelvic and chest CT, bone scan, and physical. We left and went home Monday evening not knowing the results. Dr. Cohen called Tuesday evening while I was still at work and Jeff was right beside me. She said that everything was okay! Praise the Lord, forever more. All of his scans were fine, but they want us to come back in three months instead of six. People have said, it always comes back, but they don't understand the power of our Lord and Savior, Jesus Christ, according to God's will. Someone said, you pray, and when you know your prayer is in God's will, that prayer will be answered! No matter what everyone else thinks, we're looking to almighty God, yesterday, today, and tomorrow.

I mentioned the leaf of mother and daddy's tree. Let me explain. When winter came, leaves on the trees fell off, except one leaf on the upper tree next to the road. My dad did not trim this tree because of its one leaf this year. He said this is what happened. All the leaves withered and died, turned brown, and fell off. But this one leaf, withered and brown, stayed on the tree, twisted and blown by the wind day after day, but it clung to the tree and never did it fall off. The leaf became a sign. Each morning my mother and dad would look at the tree. The leaf was always there, worn by the weather and wind, but it hung on. And Praise the Lord, Jeff, like the leaf, withered and worn by the suffering and trials of life, clung to that hope, that tree of life, the bright and morning star, our Lord and Savior, Jesus Christ. Never did he give up, and he stayed unmovable. Thank you, Lord. We believe the leaf was another sign from God, along with the oil cloth, that we must have patience, trust in Him, wait upon the Lord. Everything would be all right. The Lord has answered that prayer. We just want to serve Him. What is your will in our lives? Let us seek that will, and trust in Him for guidance. I love Him, He knows our hearts! He can look inside.

Lord, I just want to say thank you, Lord, for your blessings on me. Let us never forget what mighty power we have seen at work in Jeff's body and in our lives.

I still pray for Jack. Now Roger wants to be part of our family. O Lord, I seek your will again. Please don't get tired of hearing from me. It seems I have to ask Him something every day. But He is my best friend. You can talk to Him anytime!

I want to write about Roger next time.

I close with a thankful heart and a prayer that God will lead, guide, and direct each one of us.

Thank you, Lord!

In God We Trust.

✝

December 2, 1985

Well, time goes on. I never realized how quickly until last year. I'm sitting here by myself. The kids are at Christmas play practice. Praise the Lord! They could be involved in something else, but I pray they will always remember these times in their hearts.

I really have a hard time writing right now. I think back to last year, and my heart aches. Tears come to my eyes, and I get a lump in my throat. But, praise the Lord! He sees us through it. We have to go back to NIH December 29 for Jeff's test. We're looking to our Lord and Savior Jesus Christ, who sits at the right hand of God, making intercession, voicing our petition to Almighty God, for the results of his tests. I've been praying for Jeff to gain weight and he now weighs 132 lbs. Praise the Lord!

Last year, I went to the Christmas play by myself to watch Anita. I cried through the whole thing, thinking Jeff should be in the play. Instead he was home sick and suffering. It nearly tore my heart out. He had just had bone marrow storage and chemo. But like I said, a year has passed. The Christmas play this year is called, "The Broken Staff." Anita plays Miriam and Jeff is playing Joshua. Praise the Lord! My heart sings remembering how sick and how ill Jeff looked last Christmas. I remember thinking and praying, *"Trust in the Lord, Linda, wait, be patient, he will be better. He will look and feel better."* And now, oh Praise the Lord, he's gaining weight and he's got the prettiest curly hair you ever did see! Oh, how I love Jesus! He's going to take us home someday. Just think, to see Him, bow at His feet, and thank Him personally, just like talking to a friend. We just can't comprehend it, to say thank you, Lord, for so many blessings, even through the suffering and most of all, His sacrifices, His death, our salvation and home eternal to come!

Many things have changed in the last two years. Jack walked out of our lives, and Roger and his family came into our lives. I wonder why. I can't understand it. You know, I loved Jack, I really did; and even as I write this, he is sitting over at his mom's. He came in on a business trip. It's like he was never a part of this family. He's the kids' father and was my husband for seventeen years. What happened? I never stopped loving him. When and why did he change so much? I guess I sort of know the answer to that question. He's remarried now to Karen somebody. I don't even hate her. She doesn't know everything, and I wonder what kind of relationship they have. His new life and lifestyle surely meant more than me or the kids. Jeff's illness seemed to bother Jack, but he always seemed to be able to put it aside to satisfy his needs. Well, I don't know how I really feel. I know aside from all the hurt and anger, I do care, and I guess I always will, but I don't know what else to do now but just to leave it at the Lord's feet and ask His guidance.

As I mentioned, Roger and his family have been coming in quite often. We went to Ohio for a weekend too. I'm beginning to really miss Roger. Am I really falling in love? Is it the right thing to do? I feel there is something the Lord wants me to do, and that is what I want to do, for His glory, that it might lead someone to Him, to help someone depend on the Lord. I know I would not have been able to survive last year had it not been for the Lord. His grace is sufficient. He will never leave us nor forsake us.

What is your will, Lord? Roger wants me to marry him, but I cannot right now, for a lot of reasons. Do I really love him? We have a lifetime of family, friends, and job here. I just can't jerk the kids out of school and take them to Ohio. I know for right now, Roger and I will lead separate lives. But we have a good time together, Roger and I, the kids. Maybe the Lord sent them our way. Roger surely has helped us and brightens our days. Thank you, Lord, for a special friend when you need it!

I've had a little trouble with some of Jack's family. I try to ignore it, the hurtful remarks. They haven't been very friendly, but I just pray for them. I don't understand why they (Jack's mom especially) say some of the things they do. It hurts, but help me to pray and forgive.

Well, I better go for now. A big season is approaching, the Christmas season. Let us take time to remember and thank our Heavenly Father. We're looking to Him. Hear our pleas, dear Heavenly Father. Oh, how we love thee. Help us to know and do Your will.

"In God We Trust"

✝

March 15, 1986

Time has flown by. The last time I wrote it was December 2, 1985. Well, a new year has come in. We went to NIH on December 29 for Jeff's tests. Praise the Lord, everything was fine! Thank you, Lord!

Well, it has been a year. Jeff started his intensive treatment a year ago. Oh, how he suffered. It has taken a year for him to really recuperate. He's gaining weight, and he looks so good! The Lord touched his body. I feel it in my soul. How can I thank Him? Please, Lord, help me to search and know your will. On March 26, we will fly back to NIH for his tests again. We go trusting in the Lord and thanking Him for his healing hand and kind and tender mercy.

It has been a good year, a very busy year. Anita's in the band. Jeff was manager for the basketball and football teams so we were very busy. Anita is not really dating anyone right now, steady that is. Jeff likes a girl named Shawna, I think. O Lord, I pray that they will both find someone who will serve thee, with them. That is my prayer, that they will always serve thee.

Well, Roger and I are not going to see each other anymore. I would be relieved if I weren't worried about him and the things that I found out about him. I care for Roger, but I didn't want to marry him. He was really pressuring me to marry him, but somehow, I just knew it wasn't right. Now I know it can never be and I can't explain, the secret I know in my heart, has to remain there. I can't tell the kids or anyone the real reason we're not seeing each other, so I hope they understand it is the best thing for all concerned.

So from here, what? I don't know, but I know Who holds the future. It is, "In God We Trust."

✝

Sunday
May 4, 1986

I don't know where to start. My heart is so heavy. I haven't been able to write or hardly even read my Bible or pray. Although I pray constantly in Spirit. I'm sitting here in a hospital room at NIH again. Jeff is getting chemotherapy. Jeff has relapsed, a malignant tumor in his lung, left lung. How could this have happened all over again? Why? He was looking so good, is looking so good. Gaining weight, no pain, and then this. So he's suffering all over again. His life is threatened once again. I'm only doing now, that seems about all I can do. It's like getting so close to triumphant joy, victory, almost across the finish line of a big race, only to get knocked back and lose the race. But I know the battle, the war, is not over. Satan and sin may have won one battle but not the war. We're not giving up. Through Christ Jesus I still believe and hope. I know everyone here thinks Jeff will not survive, but Almighty God has the final answer. I believe God's words and promises. I know it looks bad, the worst, but with God, nothing is impossible. The burden seems almost too heavy to bear. Jeff suffering all over again, Anita left at home, but Jeff has shown so much faith through this.

He said, "Mom, don't worry about it. I didn't worry about it the first time, and I'm not going to worry about it now." He said he'd prayed about it. When I told him the biopsy was positive, he was angry. At no one, just mad. He's only sixteen, an age when he should be having a good time, girls, dates, cars, but not so, instead, away from home, seriously ill, fighting to live. Oh God, what does it all mean?

I thought and felt so sure it would not come back, I trusted and prayed that not one cancer cell would be left in his body. Evidently, that prayer was not answered. So, what do I do now? Satan says forget it all, what good did it do? But in Jesus's name, I rebuke Satan. I still love, trust, and pray to our Heavenly Father. I still believe Romans 8:28, Hebrews 13:5, all the other scriptures. Although my heart breaks, as only a mother could know, I'm still trusting in the true God who has all power and asking for strength for Jeff, for me, for Anita, for all of us!

They say we might be able to get some or all of the treatment at home. I ask God for guidance for the decisions that have to be made.

Anita is visiting Jack this evening, I think. He wants her to spend the night. I don't know what she will do. She says she doesn't want to hurt me. Oh God, please help me to forgive. I became so angry when this happened again, I told Jack, he and Karen should be able to figure out why Jeff is sick. SIN! I guess it was a pretty cruel thing to say.

Well, I have to go. Jeff is not feeling well. His neck is hurting. Please, oh God, please help him through this and give him strength.

In God We Trust!

✝

Monday
May 5, 1986

It is Monday morning, 9:15 a.m. Jeff is still sleeping. His neck has been really bothering him. When he awakes, I pray it will be better. He has a bone scan today and we will find out the results of all his tests. In God, We Trust.

Hopefully, we will go home tomorrow. I'm afraid, and I ask God for courage, so much to think about, counts being checked, fevers, more chemo, so much, we need your strength Dear Lord.

I need to work. I have very little sick leave left. But I don't know how much I'll be able to do. I leave that in God's hands. The school is planning a ballgame and a dance for Jeff. We are so thankful for friends and God's family. Our church, how can we ever thank them?

Dr. Barrica just told me, Jeff, they think, also has a tumor (small) in his right lung, plus the bigger one in his left lung. Oh God, we pray and ask again, in faith believing for His healing touch. Again, God says wait. We're waiting for a miracle. Help us to praise thy name.

Jeff is awake. He's eating Jell-O. He's feeling some better. As far as we know, we fly home tomorrow. Jeff's bone scan is at two-thirty, injection, scan at about two. *In God We Trust* it will be negative, his lung biopsy and bone negative, too.

In God We Trust.

†

Sunday
June 1, 1986

Time seems to fly by, it's like we're caught up in a whirlwind. Hospital, doctors, Maryland, work, school, church, although I've missed a lot of church lately, but my heart is still there. Pleasant Hill Baptist Church, it's been my life, a big part of our work for Christ. Has it meant something for you, Lord? I wanted it to and still want it to. But then I think of all that has happened. Jack leaving, the terrible, heartbreaking truth. Jeff sick, and someone, I believe Margaret said, "Linda what have you done wrong?" She was only kidding but I guess I've asked that same question. Do other people think it? I know I'm not perfect, I am as filthy rags, but the Lord washed white as snow! Praise His name forever! But I feel in my heart the Lord is trusting us with this burden for a reason, and Jeff is so strong in will and faith in God, is trusting Him, too. Anita hurts too, but she still has her faith.

Thursday night, our pastor, Lawrence Dailey, and all of our deacons (the elders) came to our house, upon our request, to anoint Jeff with oil and pray in Jesus's name for Jeff's healing. Lawrence dropped the oil on Jeff's head, and then they all laid hands on him. Then we sang Amazing Grace. Harry Stratton shouted, everyone cried, Anita too. How wonderful is our Lord, His kind and tender mercy. HOPE, our precious Savior and Almighty God has given us. Thank you, Lord.

✝

(Thursday
May 29, 1986

This was the first anointing with oil service ever held by Pleasant Hill Baptist Church. The oil is now at church, the first drop from this bottle was put on Jeff's head. But like our pastor said, there is no virtue in that oil or themselves, but the POWER of Jesus' name.)

Without Him, we could not make it. My human weakness would overtake me. Evil forces, are always present. It seems Satan has tried so hard in the last two or three years and now, to make us give up, it's like he'll stand right in front of me and say, "Now look, where is your God? Your husband left you, your son is seriously ill, you have very little money. You yourself don't feel well, high blood pressure, my car even breaks down often." I came home from the hospital with Jeff and found my refrigerator had gone bad and I lost all my food, frozen meats, everything, and it's like Satan is standing there laughing, saying, "I told you so. There's no use serving your God." But I rebuke Satan in Jesus name, His sweet name, to leave me alone, and it will ease for a while. God gives us strength to go on.

I don't by any means, really understand all this, but I am still trusting in the Lord. We probably will go back to Maryland this week for chemo if Jeff's counts are up, they're going to cut his dose, so he won't get a fever every time. He spent eleven days in CAMC with a fever and no WBC. They're going to do another scan soon. I believe the tumor is gone. The Great Physician is at work, Praise his Name! *In God We Trust.*

†

Sunday
June 8, 1986, 9:30 a.m.

Well, we're at NIH, room 247. Jeff is still sleeping, and I'm sitting at my bunk at the foot of Jeff's bed. We've been here since Wednesday. We had to spend Wednesday night at the motel. We got up here, they started his IV, and then we found out his counts were only 1,320 ACC, and it has to be 1,500. So we unhooked, went to the motel, came back Thursday, Friday, Saturday and will get it this evening at six o'clock and Monday evening. As far as we know, we will fly home Tuesday. Jeff wants to fly home on the ten-twenty-five flight so he can go to school. It's the last day of school.

They did a chest X-ray Wednesday and compared it to an X-ray that was made before his first chemo treatment. The doctor and radiologist say it is half smaller in size than before. Praise the Lord! I believe He is working through the doctors here at HIH and all of the world to relieve the suffering the human race is susceptible to. We're still trusting in our Heavenly Father, through Jesus Christ, for Jeff's complete healing. *In God We Trust*, one power, we thank Him. Also, Dr. Barriga told me his rib X-rays were normal. Praise the Lord! I'm praying it will be gone, and he won't have to have surgery. Our pastor and elders anointed Jeff with oil on Thursday, May 29, 1986.

I believe the Bible instructed us to do that…it seems the Lord directed that way, the first time in October 1984. I believe God sent the woman with the oil cloth to St. Mary's hospital and then this time we had come to NIH and brought my Guideposts magazine with me. I opened it and the first story I read was about a woman who had cancer (I remember reading her story two to three years ago about a Christmas play her family put together) and now she had relapsed, tumor to her lung, stomach. Her pastor told her about James 5, anointing of oil and she asked for it. After six months of hormone treatment, her tumor had shrunk and she was in remission. Praise the Lord! Thank you, Lord!

I listened to a church service on TV, and it really made me homesick for our little church. It's been a while, we've missed a lot lately. I can just see them gathering now, about where everyone is sitting. Oh, Lord, I pray for them and trust we will be back there, according to your will. Please watch over Anita. She's left without a home, because Jeff and I are gone up here. Please keep her safe and guide her. We miss her so much.

Well, I'm really tired this morning. I think I will rest a little now.

In God We Trust.

†

July 12, 1986

Well, we're here at NIH again. We flew up yesterday (July 11) Friday. Jeff started getting his chemo again. We will as far as we know fly home Wednesday and then go to Long Beach North Carolina with Wanda, David, Dave, and Lisa. Kristi Linville is going with Anita. I think back to a year ago today. We flew home from NIH. Jeff's check up on that Friday and then left for the beach that night at midnight with Roger and his family and Phil went with us. We'll never forget. My car broke down in Charlotte, all that, and so much has happened since then. Roger and I aren't seeing each other anymore. It was for the best I think; it just wasn't God's will. Since then, well, Jeff's relapse (March 1986), Jack's remarriage (September 1985). Jack's move back from Houston and then Jeff's relapse. Jeff has been in the hospital so much, eleven days at CAMC after the first treatment. Then nine days at CAMC after the second cycle. It has been very difficult. The last time Jeff was in CAMC we got upset with Jack. He promised to come and stay some but instead he took off for Hawk's nest with his wife and mother-in-law. Well, I got upset, and Anita and Jeff also, because I was upset I think. Jeff says he would rather Jack didn't stay. Sometimes I just don't know what to do or say. Well, anyway, Jeff was upset and he started talking. His feelings, how he would dream and wake up with tears on his cheeks, how the first time he was diagnosed he felt so close to God and how this time he would try to pray and could not. How he wanted to tell people of God and he felt too shy—and I realized he was feeling exactly what I have felt, the same closeness in Spirit the first time Jeff was sick and now this time has been different. A numbness like Jeff says, it's like when you hurt so much, you have no feelings left. Sometimes I think if I start crying, I'll never stop and I hide all my hurt to protect everyone else, including Jeff, but that night at CAMC, we both cried and cried, and I could right now even.

But in the midst of all of this, prayer has been answered. Ever since the night Jeff was anointed with oil, many prayers have been prayed, and I prayed that when his scans were done, it would just be gone and he wouldn't have to have surgery. Well, praise the Lord! The answer came. People may say, well, the chemo did it and would have anyway, but I know God's will was done and He worked such a response in Jeff. The doctors told me if Jeff didn't respond they would stop treatment. There would be nothing else. A year ago or so, this treatment was not available. Praise the Lord for such work and, I pray for this place and others, and the doctors to find a cure, all the children. On July 3, Thursday, Jeff's scan (chest and chest X-ray), were normal, no sign of tumor, and also bone scan was negative! Praise the Lord!

Oh Lord, sometimes I say, "How long?" just come quickly, because by the Word everything will be made right and healthy the way it was supposed to be. But there are many lost souls. We are in the room with Xavier Torres from Puerto Rico. It's hard to understand his mother. She has a hard time with English, but she also has faith. She told me today all there is to do, PRAY and wait! So we pray and wait, and we're still trusting in the Lord for Jeff's complete healing.

Sometimes, I think I am completely trusting Him. Even the thought of stopping treatment has flashed in my mind, but I never have felt really led in that direction. Maybe some would say if you really trusted in God, you would stop treatment. But I cannot feel led that way, I feel there is a reason why we have been here in the past and now. I pray for Jeff that he can overcome his shyness. Oh, I pray to Almighty God, give him strength and wisdom to do His will. I do believe that God has a plan for His children. The Lord gave me children, and I pray they will always do God's will.

I've questioned my life a lot lately. I look back and think did I do what I should have done in divorcing Jack? Could I have kept my marriage together if I am a sincere Christian? Then why did not my life have an influence on Jack? Maybe I want to change him for me, or I saw a side of Jack I wanted to see and not the other. I wanted and did look at Jack with trust, respect, and love. Was it my fault Jack turned to other women? I do not know. And the Bible says to pray for your enemies and forgive. Did I do that? Have I done that? Am I doing that? I need to think clearly and pray more. It seems hard to meditate now because if I do it hurts so much. The doctors say, "Well, we don't know, this treatment is new." But we believe in the Great Physician, Jesus, Our Lord, Our God, Our Creator, Our Savior, and Our soon coming King. He has all POWER, no matter what the doctor don't or can't know, it is Him (Our Savior) we trust.

Anita is seventeen years old, and sometimes I feel a little distant with her and sometimes so close. We've had to be away so much; it is very hard for Anita too. She hurts, and sometimes, there is so much attention given to Jeff, I want to give her my love and attention too; I pray for Anita. She's almost in her adult life, college, marriage. I do not know, but I pray for her to do God's will, strengthen and guide her. There are so many evil influences in this world. Please keep thy hand on her, Lord, and help me to be a better Christian mother. That is what I would like for them to remember of me, the love of our Lord. I just finished reading a book called "In His Steps." In it, a pastor asked his church to pledge with him that for one year before anyone takes an action, they would ask the question, "What would Jesus do?" It told of all the consequences which has regenerated a question that has been in my heart. I have not always done that.

Lord, I want to make the pledge, but if I truly search it out, I would have to make some changes, too, if nothing more than be the kind of mother for the kids to watch. I have always felt there is something God wants me to do with my life and that is what I'm searching for, and I pray that I will follow His will. My mind just seems jumbled right now, so many hurts, so many things I do not understand. Sometimes just so tired, sometimes like Elijah, ready to pitch your tent under the Juniper tree. But then God says, not now, just keep trusting and praying, even when we can't utter words, God hears our hearts! Praise the Lord!

In God We Trust!

✝

Monday
August 11, 1986

Well, I'm sitting on my back deck (my dad just built for me and put in a new door. He's so very good to help everyone). It has been a while since I wrote. We stay so busy. We have to go to Charleston at least twice weekly to get Jeff's counts checked. We did fly home on that Wednesday in July after Jeff's chemo. We got home at one-thirty from the airport (Anita and Kristy came and got us) and repacked and left for the beach at five that evening. Wanda, David, Dave, Lisa, us and Kristy. We drove there until 4:30 a.m. and got to where Bill, Geneva, Danny, Vicki and kids were staying. Jeff wanted to go so bad. Anita had gone for a week with Kristy Linville and her mom and dad to main Myrtle Beach, but we went for three days. While we were down there, we had to have Jeff's counts checked so we got the name of a hospital, J. Arthur Doser, a forty bed hospital, and Dr. Cazanove from NIH also called a bigger hospital in Wilmington, North Carolina (twenty-five miles away who had an adult oncologist), just in case we needed one. So on that Friday morning, Jeff and I got up and went to the hospital, but when we got there, they told us a doctor from down there had to also put in the orders. I said, but we don't know anyone. The receptionist said, "Well, there's a family practice doctor just around the corner on another street. Go see him, Dr. Gene Wallin."

So we walked around there and told the receptionist what we needed. She told us to have a seat, that the doctor was making rounds at the hospital. So we waited, and finally, they told me they called him so we wouldn't have to wait. So they gave us the orders, and we went back to the lab. We never did meet the doctor. Well, we left, and later that evening, I called the doctor to get the results. So he gave me Jeff's counts, and then he said, "How is little Jeffrey?" I said well, he's doing good, that we had been going to NIH, and he said, "That's good, that's the best place you can go. You made a right decision by going there, start at the top, taking nothing less." I needed to hear that. Sometimes, you wonder if you have made a right decision. I was telling him about the new treatment and Jeff's latest scan (praise the Lord) being negative, and he said, "Well, I believe in doing everything medically possible, but there is One greater. Greater is He that is in you than He that is in the world." And I said, "Amen, Doctor." He's the One we're trusting in.

Dr. Wallin said, "I know you feel much pain and hurt but don't be afraid." He mentioned the scripture of Jesus walking on the water and how the disciple was afraid, and Jesus said, "Be not afraid, it is I." Dr. Wallin then said, "I feel like I have known you all, all my life and we've never met except here on the telephone." He then said, "Well, I just think we should have prayer right now." Then Dr. Wallin prayed the most beautiful prayer, asking for a miracle in Jeff's life and praying for us as a family, praise the Lord! This a doctor, praying. I told Dr. Wallin that it was nice to find someone to share the faith with, and he told me if we ever needed him when we were down there to let him know. How God works! That was no mere consequence that we happened on to Dr. Wallin. There was a reason, God intended. Maybe that's what we stood in need of just then. Well, we had a wonderful time. We came back on Sunday evening. We got up Monday morning and went to CAMC and got Jeff's counts checked. Well, time passed, and thank the good Lord, Jeff did not get sick this time with a fever. They decreased his dosage to seventy five percent. They may decrease it even more, I don't know. They also mentioned radiation. We will find out this time when we go. If they want him on a twenty-one-day schedule, they will have to decrease it even more.

Well, one Friday we were at CAMC getting Jeff's counts checked, and I was on a pay phone in the lobby of the hospital talking to Geraldine Scites. Her daughter, Christina, had been in a car accident and after talking about Christina, Geraldine said, "Tell me about Jeff." So we were just talking about the beach trip, Dr. Wallin, Jeff's scans, and someone pecked me on the shoulder, and I turned around. There was a lot of people coming and going, and I don't know where this man came from, but he pecked me on the shoulder, handed me a piece of paper, and gave me the thumbs up sign and just kept right on walking down the hallway. Praise the Lord! I looked down and the piece of paper had a poem called "Accepted" and the twenty-third Psalm on it and stamped Montgomery Baptist Church, Montgomery, West Virginia. Well, again, mere consequence? I think not, a reason, God intended. There is faith in this world. God still answers prayers. He is always there. He does hear our prayers, and praise His Holy name, His power is greater than any other, and His love is all supreme!

Well, just now, Jeff is gone to football practice, the first time he has gone this year. It hurt him so much when football season started last Friday. He just went to bed, and I went off to myself to cry. I hurt so much for Jeff. Anita is involved in cheerleading now and wants to quit the band. I've talked to her, but she has completely lost interest. Seems Anita is gone so much. We're gone a lot to NIH, and she is always with her friends. She's staying with Ronda tonight so it is Jeff and me as usual. Well, I guess Anita has to have a life, too, but sometimes I just wish she would slow down long enough to enjoy being home. It won't be long until college, then it will never be the same. I love her so much, and I want her to be happy.

In God We Trust!

✝

August 16, 1986, 11:00 a.m.

Well, it's Saturday morning. Jeff is getting chemotherapy again. He started last night. He'll get it for 5 days, Tuesday night last dose. They'll unhook him Wednesday morning, we'll fly home that evening. This is his fourth cycle.

Dr. Miser told us yesterday evening they wanted him to have six weeks of radiation, which means we will have to stay up here in the motel. Well, needless to say, Jeff was upset, and it hurts me so much to see him hurt. He just wants to be at home, go to school, be football manager, go to see Cleveland Browns play. Coach Hunting is taking them in October. Instead, we are going to be here. But Dr. Miser says the tumor will come back if he doesn't have the radiation, and what's six weeks out of a lifetime? Dr. Miser says they are still looking to cure, not just treat. They have seen such good responses with the new drugs. O Heavenly Father, I pray for this place, their doctors, give them the knowledge needed to find a cure.

Besides all of this, I'm having an inner struggle, Jeff's anointing with oil by our pastor and elders. One way I struggle is this, if we believe God in fact healed Jeff, then why do we continue with the treatment? If we indeed do have faith, are we exercising it? Or are we just fooling ourselves, a cop out, like Elwood said, if it works out like we wanted (he was talking about prayer in general in any circumstance), we are thankful and say prayer was answered. If it doesn't work out, we say, well, it must not have been God's will. It is hard to understand, and the only way I can cope with all of this is to realize I don't understand. I have not the answers. How can I or anyone say why one prayer is answered and another one is not? If God is all powerful, then why do any bad things happen? Well, according to the Bible, there is always evil present, a warfare, which leads to another question, why my son? Why Jeff? Is God trying to prove something? Or is Satan trying to prove something? So many confusing questions.

I've tried to be strong, and sometimes, I feel I have no strength left. I've prayed, and sometimes I feel I can't even pray anymore. I've had faith, and sometimes, I feel my faith is so weak. I feel that maybe I just can't handle all of this and Jeff's feelings. Oh Lord, how he must hurt, anger, feeling of being cheated, and I feel that way too. He has been cheated from a normal teenage life. When his junior prom comes this spring, he will have no hair, and I pray please, God, send him someone special to care for him, love him despite how he looks. Someone for him to love, go to the prom with. Is that possible? Dear God, he needs someone so much, and I guess so do I. But I don't know what I need any more or feel. And then Anita, this is her last year at home before college, and we will be gone a lot. Anita hurts so much I know, and I love her and hurt for her too. I guess that is why my blood pressure is 178/102. I went to the doctor Thursday. He put me on another medication. I take two pills a day. He said I was going to blow a gasket if I didn't get my blood pressure down. Well, I'm tied up in knots, and I don't understand anything. But I still trust in my Lord and Savior, God Almighty. It's in His hands, and I know we have to do what the doctors say, and we are away a lot. God says wait, don't give up, and trust me, lean on me. A happy day is coming. Is that faith? Well, that's all I have right now.

In God We Trust!

✝

September 17, 1986
Wednesday

Well, it's 10:00 a.m. We've been here at NIH since Monday. At home, they told us his counts were (AGC) four thousand something. We got up here, and they were only 1408. So we've been here in room 255 for three days now waiting for his chemotherapy. If they don't go down a lot, they are going to go ahead and give him the chemo tomorrow. He'll finish next Monday; we'll go to the motel Thursday morning. He also starts his radiation tomorrow. They're going to radiate both lungs entirely. At first, I was upset they had told us five weeks just on the left lung tumor site and right lung spot. But after looking at his scans, what I understand, if I'm understanding right, what they're worried about is what they can't see, not what they see. So instead it's ten days, 1,500 rads, 150 a day. So I say thank you Lord, if they see nothing then Praise the Lord, we're still trusting in Him. Jeff has been going to school every day. We've gone out on pass every day to the mall or to the Colonial Manor for dinner.

Well, Anita is running for Miss Bobcat. I do hope she wins. She has ran for many things but has never won, so I hope she wins. But I pray for her, that she will do God's will. We just talked to her a while ago. She is at Ronda's and she has a cold. Her whole routine gets turned upside down. There's been problems, some talking. Wanda and David told me she was drinking, running around. Well, a lot of it, one of her friends, was lying to her mother about where she was going. It really hurt Anita because they accused her of doing a lot of things. I don't know. It really caused hard feelings, and I was upset too. But I guess it will work out.

There has been a change in my life, and for the first time in many years, I feel loved and cared for. You know I haven't felt this way in a very long time. Roger didn't make me feel that way. Well, Bob Swann started coming up, and it just feels so good. I told him I wasn't thinking about marriage or getting serious, but since we left Sunday, I haven't thought about much else. He fills my mind, my heart. I long to be in his arms again, to be with him. What's happening to me? I pray for Bob. He is struggling, trying to find his way or way back to the Lord. Please God, draw him, help him to turn his life over to thee. Lord, I pray I will do the right thing. I don't want to hurt him. Help me to know thy will.

Well, I do thank the Lord, His blessing toward us. The church has helped us financially. They gave us $1,100 altogether, the prayers, concern, and financial help. How can I ever repay all of this? I don't know. It's hard to be on the receiving end, but I know the Lord takes care of us and I try to work during all of this. Sometimes, I get so tired and mind jumbled, I don't know what to do. So, I just do.

Well, I'm tired. Jeff is still working on homework. I think I need to rest. Thanking you, Lord, and asking for your continued care and guidance. Thank you, Lord. "In God, We Trust."

Jeff weighs 153 pounds now. Praise the Lord!

✝

Friday
October 3, 1986

Well, we're at NIH. It's been a rough week. We went home last week-end for Homecoming. Anita was running for Homecoming Queen. She didn't win; another girl, Tanya won. It's been told her friend that works in the office put in extra votes for her, no way of proving it. I was gone and Mr. Elkins too. I really think Anita should have won, but I guess we'll never know. Anyway, Anita is our queen, loveliest of all, she is my daughter, and I love her. She is at Marsh Fork tonight at a football game. We miss her so much. She has to go with no family. Jack says he cares, but I think he doesn't, not enough. He cares more about his happiness. Anyway, we were home all weekend. Jeff's counts were down. He didn't feel well, and on Sunday night at midnight, he got a fever, and we had to go to CAMC. We were up all night in the emergency room. But the doctor at CAMC and here at NIH told us to stay there and not come up for radiation until later. So we were there until Thursday morning; they called Wednesday evening and said we should come. The doctor on 13 clinic was wrong; we should have come in after Jeff got one dose of antibiotic. Well, we flew up Thursday morning. He got radiation yesterday and this morning and will again Monday. But we will be in here until his AGC is 500 two days in a row.

It's hard being here. We get so lonely. But Jeff has been in a pretty good mood today. I'm praying his counts will come up fast so we can go home the first of the week. I pray he will stay strong in spirit and body. The Lord has been so good to us. He's always here.

He gives us hope, and it is in His marvelous, wonderful name, we trust. Give us strength, dear Lord, teach us to do thy will. We believe in God's power. We know not what the future holds, but God holds the future and our lives. It is to the one and most powerful we pray. Thank you, Lord!

Well, I think I have something else to be thankful for…and that is someone, Bob Swann. He came into my life and has shown me and given me love and caring. With Jack, I gave all the time. I loved and loved, trusted, cared and it didn't matter at all. Jack just used it for his gain, his pleasure, and now Bob makes me feel so good. I've been afraid to tell him I love him, and I think I am falling in love. Bob is just a "country boy" as he says, just plain, ordinary Bob. He doesn't put on any airs, but he fills my mind and heart, and it feels so good to be in his arms, so natural. Sometimes, it's so hard to let go, say good night or good bye. I just don't want to leave his arms, and it seems to have happened so quietly. We've only been seeing each other for about a month or little over. And now, I wonder where he's been, but maybe it's in God's timing, and I do want it to be in God's will. The way I feel, I need to say, Thank You, Lord, for sending him my way. I know Bob is not satisfied with his belief, and I pray for him that God will draw him, give him something he can feel, that he can truly serve God, and I know that we both need to serve the Lord. I miss him so much when we're up here. I look forward to seeing him again, and I can't wait to be in his arms again. What is happening to me? Time will tell…

Jeff got platelets last night, and he's been getting blood all day today, two units. It has just about all run through. He's sleeping now. It's 7:30 p.m. I get homesick and lonely, especially on weekends up here. But time will pass, and we will go home. We come and go. I don't understand all of this. I just try to cope. Without God, my Savior, I simply could not go another step. He lifts us up when we fall and gives us strength for each day. Our revival at church is coming up. I pray for it, for us, so many lost souls. We are all lost souls without the precious blood of Jesus Christ applied. I pray for Bob…

In God We Trust!

†

Sunday
October 5, 1986

Well, we're still at NIH. Jeff is still sleeping. Neither one of us could sleep last night. I think it must have been two-thirty or three before I went to sleep. I woke up about eight-thirty and finished reading my book, *No Pain, No Gain, Bruised but Not Broken* and read my Sunday School lesson. I always think of our little church back home, the people, the pastor, the building but most of all the feeling that dwells inside the building that is just a meeting place. But it holds within its walls so many memories: sadness, happiness, joy, sorrow, death and life, eternal promises to whosoever will believe Jesus's own words. Oh, Thank You Heavenly Father, for such a meeting place of thy spirit, and I pray that, the Spirit will convict and soften the hearts of all those who enter the doors.

I just talked to Bob on the phone. He is so sweet. I really care for him. I pray for him. I believe God has a special place for him in His work. I know his mom and dad have prayed for him many years, and that prayer will be answered. Is it thy will dear Heavenly Father for Bob and me to be together? I didn't know anyone could care for me like Bob does, really care. I thought Jack did, but I see now it was not like what it should have been, maybe at first. I'm not even sure now of that, but I do thank the Lord for my two beautiful children from that union. I do not believe God wanted things to happen like they have. Sin is the reason. I can't believe God would want Jack to be unfaithful because that is against God's teaching. God does allow us to make choices, and Jack did choose. I hurt so much because I loved and trusted Jack, and the marriage vow was forever, but Jack made it all null and void by his deeds. I do not understand it, and I have to realize that maybe I am to blame, partially, if only in not seeing soon enough in order to maybe have stopped it. I don't know, but Jack went his way, and now we are divorced. I didn't think I could ever love again, and sometimes, I would say, I'm better off not having someone. But then sometimes, it would hit me, just a shoulder to lean on, an arm around me, and I would say, "Please God, I need someone," and I know Roger was not that someone and then now Bob and it feels so good. I can hardly believe it, this feeling growing inside, and again I pray, Lord, I want to do thy will, and at the same time I say, thank you Lord for sending him because I do believe the Lord did send him. I never dreamed I would feel the way I do, but it's here inside my heart. Am I falling in love?

Well, we're going to be here a few days, hopefully, and I do pray Jeff's counts will come up, and we can go home Thursday. I just talked to Anita a while ago. She went to Sunday School too. We miss her so much. Dear Lord, please be with Anita and guide her. I know there are many influences and decisions she will be making, please help her to look to Thee for guidance.

"In God We Trust"

✝

Well, it's been exactly one month since I've written. We have been home, working, school, revival at church. On Sunday morning, before revival started that night, Bobby Stickler went to the altar on his own at second song we sang and gave his life to the Lord…We had a good revival. Bob Swann and I went every night. It took until now for Jeff's counts to come up. We flew up yesterday, and he got his first chemo last night. Hopefully, we will fly home Sunday. I pray Jeff will not get a fever this time. He's still has a little lung congestion where he had bronchitis last week. He got really sick with a fever of 102. I took him to the doctor; his AGC was 2,000, so they put him on antibiotic, and he started feeling better. Now he's still coughing, and they are concerned. Please God, don't let him get sick again. He's been sick so much. He needs time in between cycles. We'll be here until Sunday morning.

Well, today is Anita's eighteenth birthday. We had a family get together Sunday for her cake and everything. I called this morning and had Thompson Floral take her some flowers and balloons out to school. We're going to call her at school soon. She's staying with Ronda while we're gone. Our lives are not normal, and we are gone so much. Anita is left with no one home. Oh, that I do blame Jack for; he could have really helped during all of this but instead, he's gone. Well, I guess his new wife and new way of life means more to him than his family ever did. Father, I pray for Jack, please forgive him and I know you would if Jack would sincerely seek thee and thy forgiveness. Help me to forgive.

Well, like I said before, I think God answered a prayer and sent someone to love and that really loves me, Bob. When I say that name and think about him, I really feel love. He's made such a difference in my life. I didn't think I could ever love again nor did I think I would ever want to marry again, but I think if the timing was right and everything could be worked out, I would marry Bob today! I really do love him. All the difficult times, the hurt, Jeff's illness, worrying about that, but now I have a good warm feeling inside I never had before. That's love, isn't it? I want to be with him all the time. He's been going to football games with us too! He's been up every night that we are home. I love him!!!

We're having a hard time financially now because when I'm off work, I'm off without pay. I have bills to pay, and even though we've had help from school and church, it just goes, expenses of coming up here, going to Charleston all the time to the doctor. Well, I'm trusting in God for that too. He will take care of us. Help me to try and manage better too.

Well, I better go. I'm getting sleepy, and I am worried about Jeff's lungs. Please, Oh God, keep him safe and strong through all of this, and please watch our Anita while we're gone and I pray for Bob too. He needs thee, Lord, please draw him.

"In God We Trust"

✝

Thursday
November 6, 1986, 11:20 p.m.

Well, Jeff has had chemo Tuesday, Wednesday, and tonight. Two more days to go. Hopefully, we will fly home Sunday on the twelve o'clock flight.

They did a chest X-ray today, and thank God, it was fine. O, God, please keep him safe and strong in Jesus's name, I pray; it is in thee we are trusting. When I begin to worry and get anxious, I have to go back to that night (May 29, 1986), the elders and our pastor anointed Jeff with oil. The hope we have through thee, Lord. I know we are still continuing treatment, and there are times it would be much easier to just quit, but God gave us common sense and knowledge, and one must use it. I don't know the future and I don't claim to know it. I settled this struggle between belief and doctors, and one way was our Sunday school lesson one Sunday morning. Meshach, Shadrach, and Abednego, when faced with the fiery furnace, they could not see the future, they neither knew whether for sure they would perish in the fire or be delivered, but they stood on God's promises and purpose, and His will, and told the King that God was able to deliver them out of the furnace, but even if he did not, they would not bow to Baal. Victory and deliverance was sure only through God's purpose because even if they perished, they would be delivered from the king's hands. They did not know what would happen when they were cast in the furnace, but they did know God would deliver them either out of the furnace or into His presence. Praise the Lord! That is faith, isn't it? Oh, God help us to do thy will; there is victory through Jesus Christ. We have followed thy commandments, Lord, and you know our hearts. We love Thee; may we just be thy humble servants. I pray for Bob also. He believes in his head, but he needs to let it into his heart and to understand it is something felt, but faith, when there are no feelings, so much burden, the joy is turned into sorrow; it is still there. Maybe not those joyous shouts of the heart, but the still, quiet peace that only God can give. It is with faith, praise, and humbleness, we must turn our lives over to the Lord, realizing that God will take care of us (Romans 8:28). Sometimes, we just have to do, there are no words, no shout, just tears. But I believe and God's word promised those tears will be turned into joy, someday, in God's timing; patience, waiting, we must have it.

And you know, I feel all the last few years, the hurting, Jeff's illness, separation from Anita, Jack and losing him, and knowing the truth, then Roger. But I trusted in God and prayed to please send someone, and I waited, sometimes saying to myself and everyone else, I'm better off alone, I can't trust anyone else. I won't risk being hurt again. And then the loneliness, family get togethers, holidays and I remember praying, "Please Lord, send me a normal, healthy man to love," and then Bob started driving up on his motorcycle. We sat on the porch and drank coffee, and later, I found out he hates coffee (ha!) Then he would call and say, "Can I come up and have a cup of coffee?" So he did, and then on September 7, we had a church picnic at the lake. We sat all day and listened to gospel music while some fished, and then the next Sunday on September 14, Bob came up and brought me a flower, which is now in my Bible. We spent the day together, and that night, we kissed, really kissed, no more little pecks. Bob said, "You are making me love you," but now looking back, I know that's when I fell in love with Bob. I wouldn't tell him for a while. I was afraid and now I want to tell him all the time. We left for Maryland the next day (September 15) and I had this warm, good feeling inside and just thinking about Bob made me smile. I was in love, and now I can admit it and I say, "Thank You, Lord!" for sending him to me, and I pray we will do your will, Father. And I pray Bob will step out and claim your promises, and we may agree together to serve Thee. Please, God, draw Bob that he may feel that convicting, loving power in his life. Help me to say and do what is right.

Well, it is midnight. I'm going to close. Jeff wants me to rub his leg. Watch over us through the night. Watch over the family, everyone, Anita and Bob, and Tammy, his daughter. Thank you, Lord.

"In God We Trust"

✝

Wednesday
December 31, 1986, 7:30 p.m.

Well, 1986 is almost gone. We're here at NIH. Jeff is getting second night of chemo. We will be here until Sunday morning. This is his seventh cycle. It's been two months since he had treatment. Oh, God, help my weakness and fear. A big knot popped up on his forehead, and it scared me to death. I was really worried. Jeff said "Mom, it's probably a bug bite, what else would it be?" O, God he has so much faith. He seems happy, he smacks at me and teases me all the time. How does he take all of this? Well, God gives him strength. Jeff has a strong spirit. He's had to spend so much time in the hospital and has felt so bad. He spent nine days in CAMC in November at his sixth cycle. His counts stayed down so long.

We are scheduled to come back up February 2 for CT bone scan. We're trusting in the Lord for the results.

I guess our lives have a normalcy now, even with all of this. It's been two and a half years now. We have had to deal with all of this. In 1984, first diagnosis. In 1985, Jeff was in remission. In 1986, it brought cancer relapse to Jeff, more treatment. Jeff's life threatened again. Oh God, sometimes it hurts so much to see Jeff suffer, but yet we have a lot to be thankful for. Jeff seems to stay strong and happy, although he has days he's down. He goes to school, ball games, mall, jokes and has a good sense of humor. Anita is dating a boy named Jody now and is gone a lot. So usually Bob comes up, and Jeff is there. Bob and Jeff sometimes plays games. We rent movies. Bob has been so good for all of us. I love him. I've never had anyone to really care for me, and he does! I love him and want to marry him. But things are so complicated, the house being paid for, a lot of things. How could I ever find a love? Bob and I have something special. I feel it; he just has to touch my hand and I feel love. Is that possible? I can't wait for him to come up, and I hate it when he leaves.

Well, I don't know the future. I don't know what 1987 will hold...but God holds our future, and it is in Him we trust. His promises are in His Word, and we claim those promises. God has all power. This human side feels all the anxiety, the hurt, the worry, the doubts. God understands. He is compassionate and merciful. I feel so unworthy, so neglectful. I feel like a failure. My marriage, Jeff's illness. Sometimes I think, "what is the use?"

"Just give up," Satan says, "your life is a failure, who cares?" But the final chapter has not been written yet; in Jesus Christ there is victory!! We must press on, sometimes, most of the time, not understanding, but trusting in Almighty God, the power. This new year, dear Heavenly Father, we look to you for guidance, for strength, for your blessings. We ask. Thy word says to make our petitions known to God: wholeness and health for Jeff and Bob to find thy saving grace and to serve thee! Thank you, Lord.

In God We Trust!

Monday
February 2, 1987, 4:05 p.m.

Well, Jeff and I are sitting here at National Airport waiting for our five o'clock flight. We flew up yesterday at 4:20 p.m. flight and went to the Colonial Manor Motel. Jeff had scans done today, and his counts were too low so they sent us back home. Dr. Marrow said to call him tomorrow evening to get the results. Jeff is sitting here, reading a war book. He goes through all of this and very seldom complains. We went to 13W hospital today and visited Bruce Wiseman. He has been in the hospital for a month. He has relapsed for the third time, lung, and went back to 100 percent dosage, and it made him very sick. Also, we found out that Melissa Moore is dying; she also relapsed for the third time, and Jackie Johnson died last week. O, God, the pain and suffering, the families. Life, it seems so unfair. Margaret, my sister, works for a doctor in Huntington, West Virginia, and he told her nice people don't get sick. Oh, what an evil thing to say! So many people, nice, good people we've seen sick and dying. That doctor, if he really believes that, is way off base. He evidently doesn't know or maybe don't want to know; *Bad* things happen to good people. Good things happen to bad people. There is so much we humans don't understand, can't understand. I have to admit, and I think what it means to be wise, you know, sometimes you think, especially when you're young and some people always think that they have all the answers. Not so. Wisdom is realizing you don't have all the answers; faith is trusting in the One who does have all the answers! That is God Almighty, who sent His Beloved Son in compassion for the human race.

Who can say and I have questioned, why? Why does Jeff have to suffer? There is nothing in my mind that can justify what he has been through. But we must deal with it, live with it, trips to NIH, doctors, hospitals, sickness…death, being surrounded by illness and death, sometimes it is so overwhelming you get so tired. But, live we do and we will, live each day to the fullest, thanking God for each day, even days we think we cannot survive.

Jeff seems so strong in spirit. And I worry about Anita; she has been sick and she seems so unhappy sometimes. She and Jody fight a lot. And I think she worries about Jeff too. Anita has been very understanding, but she has been through a lot; losing a father, Jeff's illness. Dear Heavenly Father, please keep thy loving hand on her, guide her, and direct her. Well, we'll be boarding our plane soon. I don't know who's picking us up, my mother and dad or Bob. Anita went to the doctor today.

Bob, I love him. Thank you, Lord, for sending him to me. I know he needs to find thy saving grace, and I do pray for that; he is so good for all of us. The kids love him, and I didn't know what it was like to have someone to love you, care for you, someone you can laugh with, love with, that truly never wants to hurt you.

I pray we will do God's will, all of us. We're trusting in thee, dear Heavenly father, for the results of Jeff's test; our hope is anchored in Thee. I pray for NIH to find a cure, so many sick people, for the doctors to make the right decisions and for us to make the right decisions. Please be with us; I know God will always be with us. Just help us to stay attuned to thy Spirit. We need strength.

In God We Trust!

✝

Monday
February 23, 1987, 5:00 p.m.

Well, we're here at NIH again, room 255A. We've been here since Thursday. Jeff gets his last day of cycle 8 chemo tonight. We fly home in the morning on the 1025 flight (449).

Today is my fortieth birthday. Last year at this time, Jeff was still in remission, and we were home. I thought he had all this behind him. But not so, here we are again. But I know God has been with Jeff through this, his not having to have surgery, his response to the chemo, even all the fevers and blood transfusions. He remains strong, strong in spirit and body. I thank the good Lord for that. We're still trusting in God's healing hand, His power. When we got here Thursday, we saw Jerri and Ben Sebastian. Ben has relapsed for the third time; he didn't go through the intensive. He went through another protocol and then relapsed to his jaw then went through this protocol that Jeff is on now, and then two months later, Ben relapsed. All of his bones are involved now. It upset me so bad for Ben, for them; it just seems so unfair. They are good Christian people. Faith, Jeri has always said she felt God was going to heal Ben. Well, she's hurt, but she still has her faith. We were talking, tears in both our eyes for knowing at this time, it doesn't look good for Ben. You know sometimes we wish we could see the future and know the outcome. God could still heal Ben; nothing is impossible with Him and who's to say. Our human minds just can't comprehend God's plan and will. We love Ben, Jeri, and their family. They are special people; someday in heaven, Jeri and I can understand, our children can understand. Lord, please be with

Ben and his family. Jeff has four more cycles on this protocol, and oh, God, give us strength; we love you and I know you understand and feel our hurt and worry. We ask for your healing hand, and we must leave it with you. Without thee, we could not survive.

I am also worried about Anita. She is not feeling well. She had the flu, and then she had the vomiting for about five days, and Dr. Martin gave her two shots. Then I got her an appointment with a gynecologist. He gave her medicine for a vaginal infection. She went to school today and had to come home, said she was tired. I don't know what's bothering her. I know all of this has bound to have hurt her very much, and she worries although she doesn't say a whole lot. It's hard to talk about something that hurts so very deep. I pray for Anita, and I pray I can help her, whatever it is that's bothering her.

I have talked to Bob every day too. I love him, and I know God sent him to me. He loves me, and although Bob is his own man, he loves me like Jack never did. He cares about me, how I feel, what I want. He makes me feel like a woman. A woman needed and loved and wanted. I did not feel that from Jack for a very long time…a long time. I've always wanted a love like Bob gives me, and these last few months, Bob has given me something to live for. I know that sounds crazy. I have my two children, but the worries and pressure of life, Jeff's illness, has made life very difficult. I could easily say, just come Lord, then everything would be all right. But then I think about Bob and the others. Oh, please Lord, give Bob the desire and strength to take that first step toward Thee. I know he wants to, and he believes. He needs to just step out on his faith. He is so afraid he will not get anything because of the previous years. But Bob did not stay where God could use him. When you don't assemble with God's people, it is so easy to drift until you are not sure where you are. I pray Bob can find his answer, his need, and we can serve God together. I love Bob. We've known each other all our lives. Who would have ever thought we would fall in love? God does know and understands, and I think He knew we needed Bob. Robert Lee Swann, someday I hope to be Mrs. Robert Lee Swann.

There are many problems and complications…
In God We Trust!

†

Wednesday
April 8, 1987, 9:00 p.m.

Well, over a month has passed since I've written. We've been here since Monday. Jeff has had three days of chemo on cycle 9. He had all of his scans today. In God We Trust for the results. Jeff spent ten days in the hospital at home (February 28 through March 10) with fever. Since we were here, Bruce Weisman has died. Marlene, the receptionist on the thirteenth floor clinic called me at work and told me. I told Jeff after he got out of the hospital. Ben Sebastian is here now; he looks so bad. They're giving him chemo, but it doesn't look good for him. Oh, how it hurts to see him and all these others suffer. Jeff has three more cycles and then we wait… Give us strength, Lord; it is in thee we trust. Well, since I wrote last, I found out for sure what is bothering Anita. She is pregnant. I've suspected it for a long time. You know, I worried about this happening. But I thought Anita would avoid it. But Anita has suffered so much hurt. Hurt that has been buried deep inside. Anita has talked about it some. Her sense of rejection from Jack, her hurt for Jeff, her whole routine of life turned upside down. She's had to pack her bags every time we have been in the hospital and all the talk back in the fall just alienated her from all of her friends. She did not stay a night with any friends. She has been totally with Jody all the time. Jody is such a nice guy but so young. What are they going to do? My children have had to suffer in so many ways, now this. But I do pray for a healthy baby, and somehow Anita and Jody can survive all of this and someday marry and be a family. His mother will not let Jody marry Anita. I don't like the way they have treated Anita. I realize they are upset; but they shouldn't hurt Anita. I don't try to hurt Jody.

I was so hurt and upset when I found out. I didn't know what to do. I cried for two days. I told Bob about it, and he said, we would be grandmother and grandpa and we would rock it and play with it… I love him; he always makes me feel better. I believe the Good Lord sent him my way. He knew I needed someone, and Bob has a way of making me feel love and makes me feel like a woman. Something Jack just didn't do. Jack did not make me feel good about myself for a long time.

Jack called yesterday. Jeff had me tell him, he wants a car, and we ended up discussing Anita. Jack says he won't pay all of Anita's expenses because he has to pay $4,000 in income taxes. What kind of money is he making anyway? Well, anyway, surely Jody and his family will help. I don't know what their intentions are. Well, I worry about Anita. She wants no one to find out, and I know it is humiliating to her. I know that feeling of humiliation; Jack's rejection. It will be hard for Anita, especially at school. I'm not quite sure how to handle all of this, the secretary's daughter, pregnant. After all the talk, from friends, my family, this will just top the cake. How many behind our backs "I told you so?" I've heard it all the last three years, the gossip, the know-it-alls. Well, I've been hurt, Jeff and Anita have been hurt, but with God's help, we will make it.

We're still praying and trusting for Jeff's complete recovery, Anita a healthy baby, for Jody, for Bob. He wants to be saved. Lord, please help his doubts, our marriage, being a happy family, for Tammy, her happiness. Does Bob get tired of hearing all of this? I must admit, I'm tired and sometimes, especially lately, it's hard to pray. It's like being weighed down, just walking through life, doing… sometimes so burdened, and you feel like the burden is all your own that no one can share. Help me, Lord, to let others help when they can. I wonder how Jack really feels; he must hurt too. I know he and Karen need the Lord, too, but Jack always had his sight set on other things. Lord, I pray for strength; we're holding on and I pray for all these sick and suffering.

"In God We Trust!"

✝

Friday
May 22, 1987, 11:05 p.m.

Well, we've been here since Monday, May 18. Chemo Monday through today. We'll fly home in the morning. I haven't felt much like writing lately. I guess too many things on my mind. This is Jeff's tenth cycle. We come here and see so much death, suffering. Ben and Jeri are here. He is really bad. Jeri asked me to go to the cafeteria with her on Wednesday. She is really nervous now. She says sometimes she just about goes crazy. Ben is suffering, and the doctors don't expect him to get well. We sat and talked with tears in our eyes and pain in our hearts that only we can share. Jeri still has her faith; she doesn't understand, but she knows where Ben will be if he leaves this world. Jeri said just think, when Jesus sets up His Kingdom in Jerusalem, we will be there. He will have His army. Victory! Maybe the appearance of defeat now, but a vision only a Christian can see. Praise the Lord!!

Well, everyone knows about Anita now. We had to go to the welfare office and get a medical card and we'll have to change doctors. No one, Jody's family or Jack, wants to help. We'll just have to do the best we can. I need strength; sometimes I feel so weak, like I can't go on, but I'm still clinging to God's promises. Romans 8:28, Hebrews 13:5, all scripture. I'm just tired, so much to worry about. I am thankful for a lot of things each day. My children, God's love, Bob and oh, how I pray he can find that peace and satisfaction in his soul unto salvation. I love him. Well, I'll close. It seems difficult to write.

In God We Trust!

✝

Friday
July 3, 7:00 p.m.

Well, again, we've been here since Monday. Jeff's eleventh cycle. Jeff was pretty sick Tuesday but has felt pretty good yesterday and today. It's time for his last dose of chemo. Hopefully we will fly home in the morning, on the ten-twenty-five flight. I remember a year ago today; we flew home from up here. Jeff got scans and good news; tumor was gone. We flew to Roanoke airport, had dinner, and then flew on to Huntington where Daddy and Eric picked us up. I remember we were so elated with the good news. Well, it's been a year, and Jeff has one more cycle. It's been a very difficult year, flights, hospital, fevers, but we have a lot to be thankful for. Jeff remains strong and in good spirits. We have seen so many relapse here and death. Bruce Weisman died. Ben is very ill…so many others have died. We know of only one, Kevin Scarbrough, that has made it after this, second relapse; he was in remission for four years and then relapsed to his lung. It has now been one year beyond this treatment for him, and he still is in remission. It's hard to hold on to your hope when you see so much. But we still have the peace only God can give. Our lives are in His hands. Help us, O God, to be clay in your hands, the mighty potter… I know I am unworthy on my own. Without the blood of Jesus Christ applied, I would be nothing, could do nothing.

Well, Anita is seven months pregnant, and Anita and Jody get along pretty good most of the time. I pray for both of them and the baby, help us to be able to deal with all of this. I want to help Anita, but I do want her to be the mother and love and care for her child. Because I know what she would miss. There's something in caring for your child. A purpose in life, you want your children to be happy, but realizing along with that happiness, there is also pain and sorrow, but you never quit loving.

There are a lot of children here at NIH on this floor with AIDS. So sad. Good, healthy children, suffering from someone else's sin, from blood transfusions from AIDS carriers. Oh, how I pray they'll find a cure; there are good, innocent people suffering from this disease. But should we not want to make everyone well and more comfortable, even those that have brought this terrible disease to the world? But I know everything will not be made right until that day, but everyone whosoever will, the Bible says, can find forgiveness through Jesus Christ. Sometimes, everything seems so turned upside down, so many questions, no easy answers. Life, what is it? Someone said just when you think you are ready to live, then you die. You work all of your life, raise a family, maybe get ahead a little, then you stop. You are old and tired. But the meaning of life on the surface doesn't really seem worth much if you focus on that part of life, discouragement creeps in, disappointments, hurts, but there is a deeper meaning of life. You must search for it, ask questions, seek God's Word. There you will find the true meaning of life, the questions and answers; we don't just come from our mother's womb, live and then die. There is more, only through Jesus Christ. We are born naturally and live and then maybe we die but only surface life I mean, not inner life. Through Jesus Christ, we will never die, whether we die naturally or remain until His coming, for those who believe and trust, we will never die. He has promised. So we find the meaning of life to live for Him, through the good, the bad, the laughter, the tears; we live and only can we really live. It is through Him and to Him.

I thank God for his marvelous promises. I pray for my children that they'll never let the belief and faith grow cold, even with all of the problems. I know there is no other way. I think about Elwood. Oh, how I'd love to see him give his life to the Lord, and oh, I pray for Bob. I love him so much, and I know he wants to find it too. He must search, seek, look at God's Word, open his heart, and then he will find it. Jesus Christ will come in! Well, I am tired and I need to rest now.

"In God We Trust!"

✝

July 16, 1987, 10:00 p.m.

Well, we're at CAMC in Kanawha Valley, been here a week today. Jeff has had a fever a long time this time. No polys and bands. He got blood and platelets. He's tired and wants to go home. He got so upset when Dr. Starling wouldn't let him go home. I went to the mall and got him a new computer golf game, and RJ Scites stopped by to see him. It really helped for RJ to come by. He's still playing his game now, and I've been talking to Geraldine Scites on the phone. Maybe we'll get to go home tomorrow.

I feel tired and a little confused now too. Not in my faith in God and His Son, just a lot of things. Maybe I'm tired too, physically and mentally. Jeff has been in the hospital thirteen of the last seventeen days. It's so hard to explain how we really feel; hurt, anger, frustration, worry…all at the same time, but God's peace gives us grace and strength.

I know I am confused about certain things in my life, not my love for Bob. I do love him, but we need to get married, and there are so many things that hinder. I am going to have to make some decisions and I want it to be right ones, and sometimes I think, I just can't worry about it anymore. I don't want to lose Bob, but I want to do what's right. Our love has been so good and feels so good, but I want it to be in the right, and marriage would make it right. Help us, O God to work out a solution, and in asking for your help, I need to say I'm sorry for any wrong I have done. Sometimes, it seems so hard to know which way to go, but if I have done wrong, I am sorry. It has not changed the feelings of my belief, and I've got to do something to clear my confusion and feelings about my inner thoughts. Bob came into my life and gave me a deep feeling, a warmth, a love I had never experienced, and I want it to remain that way.

If Bob was a Christian, it would be much easier, but he has to want it and seek for it, ask for it. My heart's desire and prayer is that he can give his life over to the Lord, and we can be married and live the way we are supposed to. Is that asking too much? Maybe I really don't ask enough. It seems hard to keep my mind centered on God and His thoughts. My head seems so jumbled. Maybe I'm tired. I ask for thy help, Lord, and please watch over my children.

"In God We Trust!"

✝

Wednesday
August 19, 1987

Well, I hardly know how to start or how to end I should say. We flew
to NIH on Monday the seventeenth. Jeff is getting his third dose of
chemo right now of his twelfth and last cycle of this protocol. Praise
the Lord for his strength and grace that has seen us through this last
year and a half since Jeff relapsed. Oh, how long, we have waited for
this last cycle, and it is with bittersweet happiness we end this treatment. The joy of being finished and not having to come back for
treatment although, he may still get a fever and be in the hospital at
home. The anxiety of knowing the possibility of relapse and coming
back for check-up in one month; also, the sorrow at having arrived at
NIH on Monday, learning that Ben had died. I just wrote Jeri a letter
and sent them a card. Oh, how my heart aches for them. They are
such a good Christian family. Jeri had all the faith that Ben would be
healed, but it was not to be. But Ben was suffering so, and I realize
that he is now whole and healthy, but oh, to have to give them up.
We just don't understand why some are healed and some are not.
Some that are not Christians are healed. Some that are Christians
are not healed and vice versa. There are just no easy answers. But
sometimes I think, people misunderstand the word *faith*. There is a
lot of faith in the world; it doesn't always guarantee that things work
out like we want. We have to trust and believe in God's will and in
His power.

It is thee, O Lord God, I have put my trust in. I feel so inadequate sometimes, but it is through Jesus Christ that our strength

comes. So we end this last cycle with bittersweet happiness. We do say, "Thank You Lord, praise thy name. And glory and honor be unto Thee!" So many things have happened and changed in our lives in the last year.

Jeff has really grown up. Anita and Jody are expecting. They are not married, which makes it bittersweet, but yet, we are looking forward to the new life and will love it with all our hearts.

Bob came into our lives. Bob came into my life…bringing the love and caring that I knew really did exist somewhere. God sent him my way at the time when I had so much sadness in my life. But I do want for Bob, but he has to want it too, and he wants, I believe, too, to have a relationship with God. But he must first accept His Son as his Lord and Savior. I love Bob, and I want to make him happy; he makes me happy!

Well, we will be home Sunday morning. Wanda, Margaret, Annette, and Lisa are giving Anita a shower Saturday night at Wanda's house. Thank God for sisters! They've been so good to us and my mother and dad too. I also go to work August 26. A new school year. Jeff is a senior. With all of my heart, I hope, pray and trust this will be a good year, a year he can enjoy at school.

We leave behind friends, a lot of sad memories; we've lost so many of our good friends; so many memories, tears, loneliness; now looking to a new year, a new life, love, health, and most of all trust in our loving Heavenly Father that has brought us through with prayers for this place, doctors, nurses, families, the sick, praying for God's strength and help to go on. One day at a time. We love thee, Lord Jesus, realizing you first loved us.

"In God We Trust!"

†

Monday
November 23, 1987

Well, I could write forever and never fill the pages. So much has happened…but I could not write; my heart is too heavy or was. After Jeff's last chemo cycle in August, he did get a fever. But finally, all that was over. School started; we were back into the routine of things. Heather Lakin was born to Anita and into our hearts on September 11, weighing 6 pounds, 10 5/8 ounces. You know, I was so upset when I found out Anita was pregnant, not so much at her; my love for my daughter will never change, but hurt and disappointment I guess. But, Jeff finished his protocol in August. Heather Lakin was born in September. We spent probably the best two-and-a-half months than we've spent in a long time. We were home, all of us. Bob is there with us when he can be. Anita, Heather Lakin. Jody is there a lot. Sometimes, it's so hard, problems between Anita and Jody, but if it is for the best, I do hope things work out for them so they can be a family and be happy. They need to keep their faith and stay close to the Lord and church.

But on October 15, we flew back to NIH for chest X-ray and on Friday, October 16, our world fell apart again. Dr. Hoki called and said there was a suspicious legion on Jeff's X-ray, left lung. I lost control. I must admit. I cried, stomped my feet in anger. It was just not fair after all he's been through. Jeff cried and said, "I just want to graduate and see Heather Lakin's first birthday." At that point, I simply had no words. How can you offer comfort when you have run out of words of comfort? When all your strength is exhausted. That is how we felt. Our faith was stretched to what I thought was my limit. I said, I must accept what I haven't wanted to accept all along. I say, why God, after all he has been through? And I say, okay, this is the way it's going to be, give us the strength to face this. For about one week, I was in a twilight zone, doing and not wanting to do. I didn't want to go to work, see anyone. I got tired of talking. I couldn't go to church. Our revival started, and it was an effort to go, but amidst all the hurting, I know deep down inside my faith was still there. I felt God was so far away, where was He? I was hurting so bad, but I know He was always there. How could I have gone to work, to the revival or anything? I really was not functioning on my own strength. But after a couple of days, Jeff just got up, went back to school, basketball practice and whatever. I said, okay, this is the way we handle it… keep going, live every day as normal as possible. Finally, the doctors called; they had to decide what was best. They called saying surgery needed to be done on November 19. This brings us to now. We got here last Wednesday, leaving family and friends behind. Jeff was told by the surgeon on Wednesday night, straight forward, if there was more cancer in his lungs, they would just sew him up. There was no effective chemo to offer at this point. Dr. Pase, said this is Jeff's chance to live. I asked Dr. Pase how he would know if his lungs had cancer, and he held up his hands and said, "These fingers right here," if more cancer, surgery would not take place, and praise the Lord, when he went in, his left lung was clear. He told us he felt very good about the operation. That he thinks he got it all. Oh, Praise the Lord, everything looked so down. Now they're telling me he has another chance to live. Oh, ye of little faith, was that me? Well, maybe, but we were still trusting in our Heavenly Father, so hopefully we will be flying home Wednesday morning on the ten-twenty-five flight. Thursday is Thanksgiving! Thanksgiving! Thanksgiving!

Thanks be unto God for His marvelous mercy and power! So once again, we go home with thanks and praise to our Father and hope in our hearts. It is still to Thee we look and trust to the future. He will never leave us nor forsake us (read Hebrews 13:5); even when we can't seem to feel or feel forsaken, He is there! He gives us strength when ours is gone…He gives us peace when there is none…He gives us hope when all hope is gone. He gives us always His Love and comfort. He gave himself so we could have all this and promises yet to come.

Jack, Karen, and his mom came up here on Wednesday evening and stayed until Sunday morning. I hardly remember Wednesday and Thursday. It made it hard having them here. They all three came in and sat down on my bed. I had to sit up all day in a chair, and they just sat there and watched him. As soon as they would leave, Jeff would perk up and want to play cards or something. But I just dealt with it. I really didn't have much to say. I listened; here they sat, Jack, the woman that tore a home up, and his mother. Mrs. Salmons kept saying I wouldn't have let you go through this for nothing, and I said, "Well, we've been through a lot by ourselves for three years," and I said, "Let me tell you something, if I had insisted, Bob and my mother and dad would have been here but the money they would have spent in motel rooms or plane fare, they're giving us to live on." Mrs. Salmons really loves Jeff and her intentions are good, but it did not help me having them here, but if it in anyway helped Jeff, then it was all right. That is all that matters. Well, I'm really tired this evening, so I think I'll close with a thankful heart and prayer for all these sick children and doctors that they will continue to work to alleviate some of the suffering in this world. There is so much to pray for, but God also knows what we need even before we do. Thanksgiving! Thanksgiving!

"In God We Trust!"

✝

Friday
March 25, 1988

Time flies. We're sitting at National Airport waiting for our plane to go home. We flew up yesterday, a repeat of scans done in February. We came December 15 and again on February 15. A "hot spot" as the doctors call it showed on his bone scan, and there are subtle differences in the surgery rib site. So all over again, hurt, frustration, worry gripped us; we all cried. Anita laid on Jeff and cried, "It's not fair, just not fair." Why can't things be normal? Jeff said things haven't been normal and never will be, and I guess he's right. When you've been through what he's been through the last four years, cancer, the normalcy of life is gone forever. But after a few days, like before, we adjusted, put the worry in the back of our minds, went on with our lives, work, school, church. The doctor wanted us to come back up here March 15, last week but Jeff said, "No, we're going to the State Basketball Tournament and I want to be there." So I called NIH, and they said okay, let him go, enjoy; one more week won't matter. Well, Hamlin not only went to the State Tournament, we were state runner up Class A! Which then brings us to now…

Dr. Hoki was able to get the initial reading by the radiologist, no change chest X-ray or chest CT. Praise the Lord! *No change*…at this point that is good…great news. They will read the bone scan Monday. Oh, I pray in Jesus's name the bone scan will be good. Jeff looks so good. Six feet one inch, weighs 175 pounds. He's got prom, senior trip, graduation coming up…O, Lord, what plans do you have for him? He has a story to tell. I pray for Anita and Jeff and myself and baby Heather Lakin to let the Lord use us. Sometimes I feel like such a failure, but the good Lord knows every heart, and I do love Him. I pray for Bob to find salvation.

Well, Jeff said, when I told him about his CT and chest X-ray, "I wasn't worried, there's no use in worrying about it." He's been through this so many times. Thank you, Lord, for his inner strength that I know comes from you. Baby Heather Lakin is six months old, growing, has brought so much love and smiles to us. Anita and Jody have been broken up since before Christmas. I don't know, please be with them Lord, that they may always look to Thee.

Well, it's almost time to board the plane. We will talk to the doctor on Monday. It is in Thee, dear Lord, we trust. Thank You, Lord, for thy tender care and mercy. (We also found out that Raymond Emerick died last Friday.)

"In God We Trust!"

✝

Wednesday
June 22, 1988, 3:30 p.m.

Well, once again we are at National Airport waiting to catch Flight 303 home. Three months have gone by, three glorious months as after the last trip up here. The news was good; the hot spots they saw, surgical scar, unchanged, hot spot on upper rib, less. Dr. Hokin said tumor does not get less, tumor does not go away. Praise the good Lord, relief flooded our souls. Since then, Jeff has been enjoying his senior year. A senior trip to Myrtle Beach and at prom, he and Hope Ginn were elected Prom King and Queen. Jeff and his date Angela Slone danced. After prom was at Dunbar. Graduation was the next weekend. Jeff received the Presidential Academic Fitness Award for extraordinary effort to achieve academic fitness. He graduated with a 3.2 average. He now weighs 193 pounds; he's been off treatment since last August. Surgery in November on ribs, so that brings us to now. We are supposed to talk to Dr. Aplin Friday for the results. It is *"In God We Trust."*

Heather Lakin is now nine months old. She says grandma and is walking. She is her sweet, lovable self. I love her like my own. Anita is a good mother; she gets up at night with her. She misses her mama when Anita is gone. Anita and Jody were back together since Mother's day and now trouble. I just don't know what to do about those two. They have to work it out. But they seem to make each other miserable. Will Jody ever grow up? He makes life miserable for Anita. I pray for them.

Bob is so good to us. He tries to really help me, and I believe he really does love me. I thought Jack did, but things are so different between Bob and me. It is good, and I pray for Bob. He knows he should give his life to the Lord, but he just won't step out. There's a lot of things I guess we need to work out, marriage, but we're trying to be patient. I love Bob, and he makes me very happy. I have fun with him. I enjoy being with him.

Well, it won't be long till we board. It's very hot, 100 degrees here; it's even hot in the airport. We have been so busy, school, church, Bible School. We had twenty teenagers in class. I taught the teenagers for the first time. I'm used to younger, but I enjoyed and did learn myself.

Life is fast, but God intended for us to be busy. Even when found with difficulty and uncertainty. I learned in Bible school from studying about Paul and his conversion what he suffered. Uncertain future but he continued, even while imprisoned, "business as usual." He continued preaching and praying.

Whatever God's plan for us to do, no matter what, we should continue "business as usual." That makes life worthwhile, eternal hope and peace through our Lord and Savior Jesus Christ. It is "In God We Trust!"

†

Tuesday
July 19, 1988, 8:50 a.m.

Well, I don't think I can write much. Jeff has relapsed for the fifth time, spot on both lungs and right rib. Can't operate, no radiation, he's had too much already. When we got the report, I cried and cried. Anita cried. Jeff just said, "Well, shit," and went to bed. But after ten to fifteen minutes, he started asking questions, where was it? He said if they told him nothing or chemo, he would take the chemo. Jeff also said if he has to leave, he has a better place to go. Only God can give one that kind of peace. Praise the Lord for that, and I feel God understands. He's eighteen and he wants to live and he will fight to live, so will we, whatever we have to do. I only hope and pray that he will respond to this treatment. We have to live with hope; we can't live without that, and each day gives them more time to find a cure. God's work is here, helping the sick, God's love... (I called Jeri Sebastian today, Ben's mom. Ben died a year ago. They are Christians, and they said they would pray for us.)

Since Jeff's relapse, I guess I've sort of felt numb. Four years of fighting, praying. It is so frustrating and sometimes I think how can I pray for something I've prayed so many times for? I feel tired and frustrated, human emotions, but beyond this, I feel hope, I still pray. God knows my heart. There seems so much to pray for, so many sick, family, friends, Heather Lakin, Bob. Oh, how I pray he could find salvation, feel, experience God's salvation, freedom, love, hope... Dear Lord, please even when I am tired, know my heart's desire. It is *"In God We Trust!"*

†

Thursday
August 18, 1988, 7:25 a.m.

We are sitting at Washington National Airport for our flight home. How many times have we done this? I don't know. We flew up Tuesday morning, and they told us they were reducing his 6MP dose to twenty-four-hour infusion because his Bili Reuben (liver function) went up to 3.0, and they don't want to cause him liver problems.

His chest CT showed maybe stable or slight progression of tumor. They can't really tell. We're still praying, trusting that Jeff will respond to this treatment. He is still very strong and looks really good. This thing called cancer is still trying to take over his body, this disease is so hard to understand.

Jeff has a girlfriend, Missy Mullins from Hurricane. They have exchanged rings. She is a very pretty girl and sweet. I thank the good Lord; she has been so good for Jeff and his friend Kevin Byrd, is a true friend. May God bless him. Anita and Heather Lakin are fine. Anita is getting ready for Marshall. Heather Lakin is growing and learning something new every day. She is so sweet, a blessing from heaven.

Well, I'm very tired, we've still got about an hour before flight time. We have to come up again in about three weeks for scans and 6MP. I'm still praying for Bob. I love him very much.

In God We Trust!

†

Friday
September 17, 1988, 7:19 p.m.

We're sitting in the lounge on the fourteenth floor of NIH. We've been here since Monday, September 12, getting new treatment.

It's so hard to write anymore. I guess the words just don't come easily. Life has became mind boggling and overwhelming at times. The 6MP Jeff was on didn't work. The tumor in his left lung doubled in size (about one inch now). They stopped it; now he is on Pertrixin. Jeff is the first pediatric patient, the first Ewing's patient to be treated with this drug. It has been tried on adults with other types of cancer. Some responses in colon cancer patients, but since Jeff is first, they simply do not know, so we're still hoping and praying this is the answer, this is the way to rid his body of his disease. Jeff's body is so healthy; he looks great! This cancer just won't go away. I tell you, you'd think we would be used to it, but it doesn't get any easier. Jeff keeps fighting; we keep hoping and praying. Please God, let them find a cure. I've wondered and asked so many times, why? Why did this thing have to happen to Jeff? As Jeff says, "why anybody?" Well, I do not claim to understand, but we are still trusting in God. He has all power. Jeff tells me, "Mom, if they tell me I'm going to die, it's okay. I know I have a better place to go, and I won't be sick anymore." What faith! Jeff is at peace with dying, but he wants to live; he will not give up. He told the doctors, "I will not quit." Dr. Balis said, "Then we won't either." I thank God for this place. So many would not have any place to go, no one to really help; truly this place is God's handiwork, to help make things better.

Jeff is a true-to-life *hero*. Battles are fought on the battlefield during a war by courageous, brave people. Well, it's no different; only that Jeff's enemy is inside his body trying to kill him, just like bullets, weapons, the enemy. Jeff hasn't retreated; he's fought long and hard. He's suffered pain, physically and mentally. Loneliness from being away from home and family, but he has stood strong. Only that strength has come from the Lord; Jeff has inner strength and peace that no matter what happens, it will be all right. I think this gives him the courage to fight, and Jeff always manages to lift your spirits. He also has a good sense of humor, always joking, his way of saying, "I love you, Mom." It keeps me going.

Anita is still going to college. Heather Lakin is doing fine, but Anita says she has cried all week. She goes to my room and Jeff's room and stands and cries. She's a blessing straight from heaven. I know the circumstances between Anita and Jody, and I don't understand and I hate it that Jody does not have the relationship of father-daughter with Heather Lakin. But that is the way it is. Hopefully it will not hurt Heather Lakin, and we've seen so much hurt already. Heather Lakin knows she is loved. I just want what is best for her and Anita. I pray Anita will find someone to love and care for her, really love her. It seems that is so hard to find any more. We live in a self-caring world; true love is hard to find. Jeff is still dating Missy Mullins. She seems to really care for Jeff. I know he does for her and I hope they don't hurt each other. But I thank the good Lord for her. She truly is good for Jeff. And I pray for Kevin Byrd too. He has been such a good friend to Jeff. Well, we've been here at the hospital since 8:00 a.m. (twelve-hour blood draws). We've been in the motel all week. He gets one more stick at nine and then we can unhook and go back to the motel. Our plane leaves National Airport at 8:35 in the morning. It's always so nice to go home. I miss Bob too. He is so good to me, just in lots of ways, that I know he really loves and cares about me.

Bob wants to be saved. We're still waiting for this event, praying. Please help him, Lord.

Well I will close. We're tired. We have another hour to go. My prayer is for this treatment to work. He can take it orally, three pills a day, what a relief after what he has been through.

"In God We Trust!"

✝

October 27, 1988

It is with a simple "Thank You" dear Lord, we go home from NIH again today. We really needed the news we got today. The results of Jeff's test done yesterday, bone scan, nothing—arm and leg fine, chest CT, stable, maybe a nodule a little smaller. The doctors said, "We did not expect this, with a phase I drug."

I asked, "Are you saying he responded?" and answer was yes, definitely stable. We have hoped and hoped. Each time it got so hard, then today, we hear this! Halleluiah! Praise to our good Lord! I just can't find other words right now. I have so much in my heart, mind... so we go home with Peritrixen to start in the morning, and we will return Monday night to get twelve-hour blood draw on Tuesday, and then we go home. We will come back November 21 for next treatment. Prayer has been answered! Praise His name!

I called Anita. Thank you Lord, I don't know what to say except:
Thank you, sweet Jesus!
Thank you, dear Lord!
Thank you, Heavenly Father!
Praise His name!!
In God We Trust!

†

December 9, 1988

Well, we're in the hospital at CAMC Kanawha Valley. Fever, mucositis, feet raw, and peeling from Peritixin. Jeff has had four cycles of this drug, and it has been considered stable disease, cancer still there, just not growing since September. We go every three weeks to NIH for chest CT and decision whether to continue this treatment. We are thankful for the results, but the pressure is very difficult, the waiting, but what else is there to do? Live with it; enjoy our times together, the bad and good. Life is very busy. Jeff's illness, Anita in school, Heather Lakin, Bob, work, church. I have only twelve days sick leave left. I don't know what we'll do when my sick leave runs out. I don't worry about it; we've got too much else to worry about. Now Jack is taking me to court; he wants relieved of all responsibility. He doesn't want to pay for the house anymore. Why now? With all we're dealing with, he does this. He and Karen probably make $100,000 a year. I make $14,000. I don't know what is going to happen. I get so tired. I actually got sick when they delivered the paper to school. What kind of person would do this? His own family, his own kids. We need help, not this. But we are still looking to our Heavenly Father. I don't understand this, but there is a lot I don't understand.

Jeff has been so sick. Dear Lord, we need your help. Anita is seeing someone new. He's some older. I just hope and pray she will find someone to care, really care and love her and love Heather Lakin too. She is so precious! Well, hopefully, we'll go home tomorrow, been here since 2:00 a.m. Wednesday morning December 6. We go back to NIH December 18. Please, we pray for good results. It is with thankful and prayerful heart I close.

In God We Trust!

✝

Tuesday
April 4, 1989, 7:00 p.m.

So much time has passed since I've written, but seems I just can't write anymore. If I stop too long, think too much, pray too long, read my Bible, it brings so much emotion to the surface. I feel as though my tears would never stop. My heart is breaking. My beautiful son is suffering. Off Peritrexin, relapse, tumors growing. We left NIH. Jeff has exhausted every protocol NIH has for Ewing's. So we're getting treatment at home now in Charleston. Dr. Starling had a protocol from another pediatric oncologist group. Ara C, eighteen treatments, once a month. It's like you don't know what to say or do anymore. It hurts too much. We are thankful for Dr. Starling, our family, our friends, people who help. Anita's boyfriend is so good to her and Heather Lakin. I pray for them to be happy, go to church, talk to and have a relationship with the Heavenly Father.

Bob and I plan to marry someday. Arb, his mother has Alzheimer's disease. So he spends a lot of time with her. He still needs to make a commitment to God. I'm still praying. We need strength from on high. It seems so much gets thrown at us, but my faith in the Lord is still there; it just seems there is so much hurt.

Jack is refusing to pay the $100 a month the family law master told him to. He's taking it before Judge Stevens. He doesn't call and see about Jeff. He tells him they will do something but doesn't show up. Oh, how could he hurt Jeff so? Jeff cried when he didn't show up Saturday. Jeff doesn't need that now; no child needs that any time.

He has hurt Anita and Jeff so much. I don't care what he does, but what he does to Anita and Jeff is what matters.

Heather Lakin is so sweet and beautiful. I tell her I love her and she says love too. She puts joy in my heart and a smile on my face. Please watch over her and keep her, dear Heavenly Father. We'll be here until Thursday morning. Jeff said this evening, "I want to go home."

I say, "Honey, I know, but we have to be here," and I hold his hand, rub his head, his back and say, "Honey, I love you, just relax," and he takes a deep breath and says okay. I rub his back and hold his hand, and I think of when he was just a little boy in my arms, rocking and feeding him. He's still my little boy, my love is the same. Why did this have to happen? I cannot answer that. We only have to deal with the way it is, all of the pain and the suffering. It can't take away our love for each other.

"*In God We Trust!*"

Anita, Jeff, now Heather Lakin, nothing can ever take that away from us. Bob Swann is a part of us now. He has been so good to us. I pray for him to make peace with God.

Go with us Lord, we need your strength. This cup we have to drink from in life is hard. I have no greatness, no magic power, just the same hurt, frustration, and agonizing pain that anyone feels when their child is suffering. I have and I am nothing, but through our Lord and Savior, we have everything. That is what Jeff needs to feel: peace, love, and hope.

"*In God We Trust!*"

✝

Thursday
August 16, 1989

God is our strength.
>God is our refuge.
>Who shall we fear?
>Oh, God, I am weak.
>And I am afraid.
>Does that speak much for my faith? I only know what I believe in my heart, and I still hold those truths that are written in the Bible, God's precious Word.
>I have failed my marriage, my children, my whole life. A divorce, an unwed mother (my daughter), my son, suffering so much with cancer. What does it all mean?
>God loves us…all things work together for the good of those who love Him and called according to His purpose. I don't claim to be perfect because I have sinned. But God is my Father. I am His child.
>The answers are far too deep, overwhelming for me to find. The suffering we have endured, that Jeff has endured. Where is the truth, the justice, the wrongs made right? That is the only answer I can find; it lies with Almighty God.
>Jeff is seriously, seriously ill. This awful, awful disease called cancer just keeps eating away at his life. All the prayers is what is so hard to understand. If you believe in the power of prayer, some say the answer comes in many forms, but when the plea, the prayer is for fighting a disease like cancer, when the answer is life or death,

no in-between, the answer is pretty clear cut...you live...or you die. How could you mistake the answer? If Jeff must die, we must see the purpose; his death could not be in vain. He is fighting with courage, patience, peace, even a sense of humor, with faith.

Even abreast his emotional human feelings of bitterness, betrayal, physical pain...Jeff fights back with quiet acceptance, love of God, and faith. The bitterness eases with tears shed, prayers prayed.

Jeff has gotten one treatment on another phase I drug Fara amp/Fludarabine. It did ease his pain some but has not stopped the spread of the disease. Jeff knows this and even without telling him. Jeff has seen so much, watched so many of his friends die. Those words between us need not be spoken...he knows.

I know what the doctor says but we still look and cling to our Heavenly Father. He is our only hope and always has been. I have no big prayer, no big words; it hurts too much to even speak. I have only what my heart speaks...prays. We need your help, O God. We are falling, drowning. Give us a miracle in Jesus's name, we pray.

"In God We Trust!"

✝

Jeff passed away August 25, 1989 at 12:15 a.m. I have not been able to write...someday maybe. Jeff's life is not forgotten. I remember. I promised him. I do not understand. It hurts so very much... The pain never really ever goes away. It is still to God we look to, cling to. Jeff is with Him now. He is well, no more suffering, but in my heart, I want him here with us...

In God We Trust!

Psalm 143:10 "Teach me to do thy will; for thou art my God: thy spirit is good; lead me into the land of up rightness."

"Our feet can walk in sunshine, our hearts can know his light. Jesus conquered darkness, His blood has won the fight!"

> And Jesus saith unto him, I will come and heal him. (Matthew 8:7)

> Ask, and it shall be given you: seek, and ye shall find: knock, and it shall be opened unto you. For everyone that asketh receiveth; and he that seeketh findeth; and to him that knocketh it shall be opened. (Matthew 7:7–8)

> And Jesus saith unto the centurion, go the way; and as thou hast believed, so be it done unto thee. (Matthew 8:13)

> Come unto me, all ye that labour and are heavy laden, and I will give you rest. (Matthew 11:28)

> For where two or three are gathered together in my name, there am I in the midst of them. (Matthew 18:20)

> With men this is impossible; but with God all things are possible. (Matthew 19:26)

> And all things, whatsoever ye shall ask in prayer, believing, ye shall receive. (Matthew 21:22)

> But he saith unto them, it is I; be not afraid. (John 6:20)

> Let not your heart be troubled; ye believe in God, believe also in me. In my Father's house are many

mansions; if it were not so I would have told you. I go to prepare a place for you. And if I go and prepare a place for you, I *will* come again, and receive you unto myself; that where I am, there ye may be. And whither I go ye know, and the way ye know. (John 14:1–4)

Let not your heart be troubled, neither let it be afraid. (John 14:27)

For in him we live, and move, and have our being. (Acts 17:28)

As it is written, there is none righteous, no, not one. (Romans 3:10)

And we know that all things work together for good to them that love God, to them who are that called according to his purpose. (Romans 8:28)

That your faith should not stand in the wisdom of men, but in the power of God. (1 Corinthians 2:5)

Rejoicing in hope, patient in tribulation, continuing instant in prayer. (Romans 12:12)

Because I live, ye shall also. (John 14:19)

We are troubled on every side, yet not distressed: we are perplexed, but not in despair; persecuted, but not forsaken; cast down, but not destroyed. (2 Corinthians 4:8–9)

I will never leave thee, nor forsake thee. (Hebrews 13:5)

And whatsoever ye shall ask in my name, that will I do that the Father may be glorified in the Son. If ye shall ask anything in my name, I will do it. (John 14:13–14)

I can do all things through Christ who strengthens me. (Philippians 4:13)

Wait on the Lord; be of good courage, and he shall strengthen thine heart; wait, I say, on the Lord. (Psalms 27:14)

Now faith is the substance of things hoped for, the evidence of things not seen. (Hebrews 11:1)

Whom having not seen, ye love; in whom, though now ye see him not, yet believing, ye rejoice with joy unspeakable and full of glory. (1 Peter 1:8)

Beloved, think it not strange concerning the fiery trial which is to try you, as though some strange thing happened unto you. But rejoice, in as much as ye are partakers of Christ's sufferings; that, when his glory shall be revealed, ye may be glad also with exceeding joy. (1 Peter 4:12–13)

Casting all your care upon him, for he careth for you. (1 Peter 5:7)

And whatsoever we ask, we receive of him because we keep his commandments, and do those things that are pleasing in his sight. (1 John 3:22)

And this is the confidence that we have in him, that if we ask anything according to his will, he heareth us; and if we know that he hears us, whatsoever we ask, we know that we have the petitions that we desired of him. (2 John 5:14)

God is our refuge and strength, a very present help in trouble. (Psalms 46:1)

What time I am afraid, I will trust in thee. (Psalms 56)

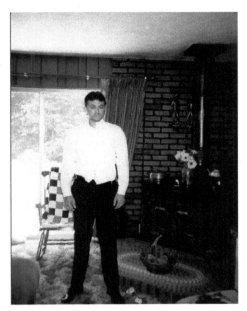

Jeffrey Salmons dressed for his senior Prom
1988. "Tall, dark and handsome."

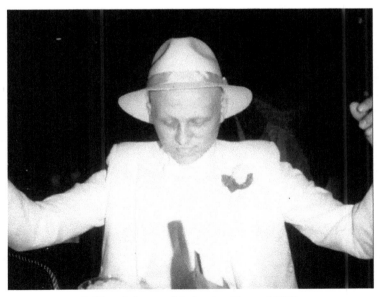

Jeffrey Salmons his Junior Prom 1987.
During treatment, no hair but still enjoying prom

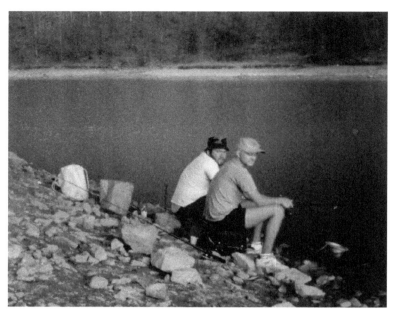

Jeffrey and his first cousin, Dave Owens fishing—they loved it!

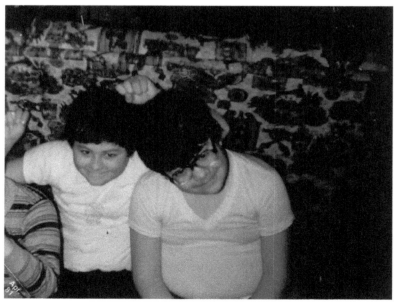

Jeffrey and his first cousin, Eric Nelson who was
by his bedside when he passed away.

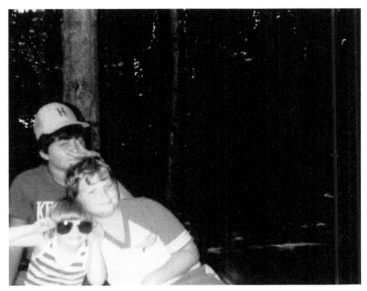

Jeffrey and his first cousins, Chris and Carrie Nelson.
He loved his family!

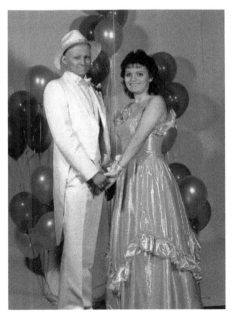

Jeffrey Lee Salmons, junior Prom 1987, pictured with
his sister Anita. He was in treatment at this time.

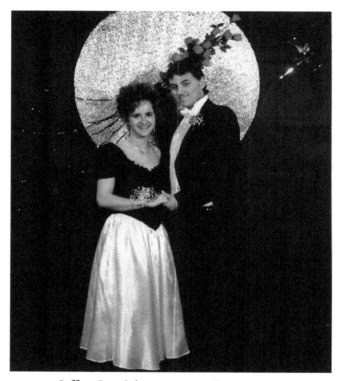

Jeffrey Lee Salmons, senior Prom 1988,
pictured with his friend, Angela Slone. He was still in
remission at this time but would soon relapse.

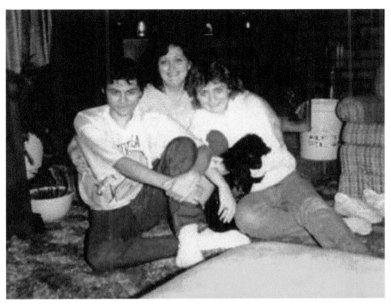

Jeffrey Salmons and his mother, Linda and sister, Anita.

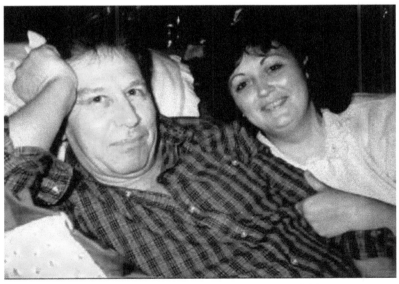

Robert Swann and Jeff's mother, Linda, who would later marry.

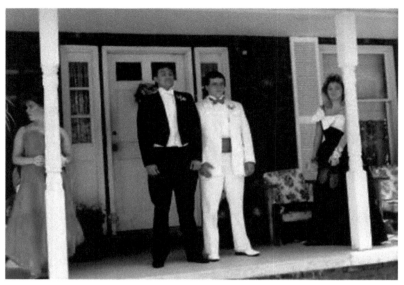

Jeffrey Salmons, his friend Kevin Byrd Prom 1988

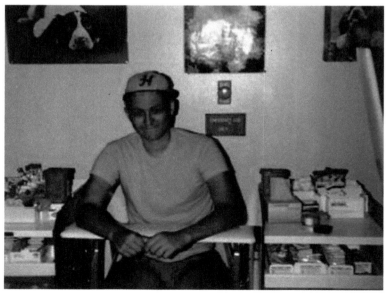

Jeffrey Salmons getting lab work done during
his treatment for Ewings Sarcoma

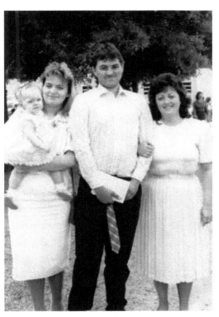

Jeffrey Salmons, mom Linda, sister Anita, and niece
Heather Lakin. His graduation 1988.

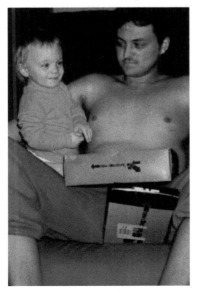

Jeff Salmons, holding niece Heather Lakin. He passed away 8/25/1989

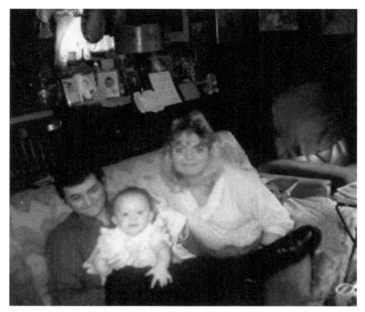

Jeffrey Salmons and his sister Anita, and his niece Heather Lakin

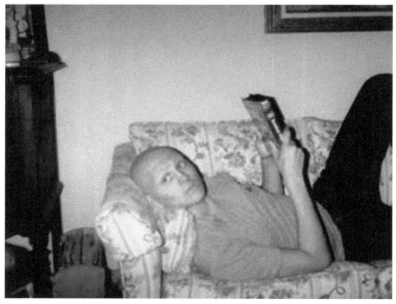

Jeff Salmons during his treatment for Ewings Sarcoma

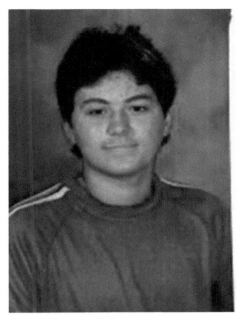

Jeffrey Salmons age 14

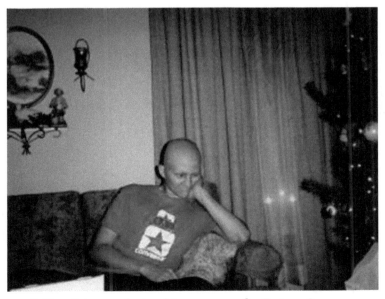

Jeffrey Salmons during his treatment for Ewings Sarcoma

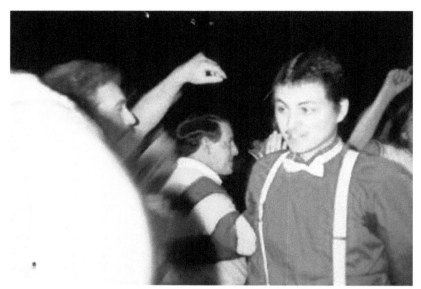

Jeffrey Salmons at Basketball State Tournament
in Charleston, WV fall of 1988

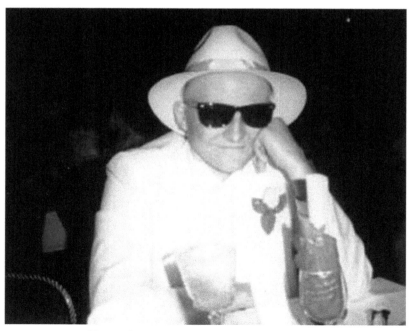

Jeffrey Salmons at prom, Hamlin High 1987.

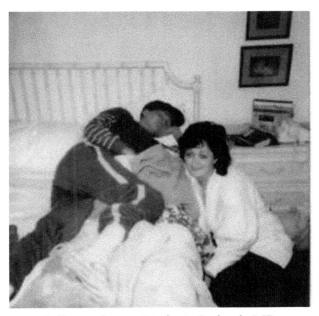

Jeffrey and mom Linda, in Bethesda MD

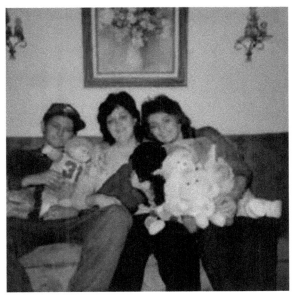

Jeff, mom Linda and sister Anita

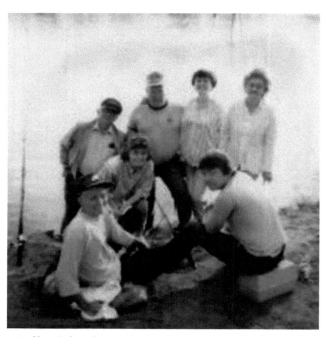

Jeff and family on the Potomac River after hospital

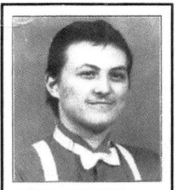

JEFFREY LEE SALMONS, born April 15, 1970, went home to be with Jesus, on August 25, 1989. Jeff loved life, his family, his friends. He loved the Heavenly Father and put his trust in Him a long time ago, although he was only 19 years old. Jeff suffered so much physical pain, but his inner strength and faith in God gave him the courage to live each day in hope; to smile when there could have been tears; to laugh when there could have been weeping; to hope when there could have been despair; peace when there could have been fear; and life where there could have been death. Jeff is now in that eternal life in the arms of Jesus with no pain and suffering, only happiness. Jeff leaves behind his mother, Linda Salmons of Hamlin; father, Jack Salmons of Hurricane; sister, Anita Salmons of Hamlin; niece, Heather Lakin Salmons of Hamlin; grandparents, Hurxel and Beulah Woodall, and Virgil and Emma Lee Salmons, all of Hamlin; a special friend, Bob Swann of West Hamlin; and many family members and dear friends. Jeff was a member of the Pleasant Hill Missionary Baptist Church, and was a graduate of Hamlin High School, where he played, and finally became manager for his football and basketball teams. Services were conducted on Sunday, August 27 by the Rev. Lawrence Dailey and Rev. Mickey Salmons. Jeff was laid to rest in Fairview Memorial Gardens, Hamlin, WV.

In Loving Memory of Jeffrey

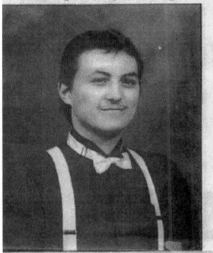

In loving memory of Jeffrey Lee Salmons who left us eight years ago August 25th. He will always be in our hearts and a part of our lives. He was a special person who brought so much happiness into our lives for those short nineteen years.

Safely Home

I am home in Heaven, dear ones;
Oh, so happy and so bright!
There is perfect joy and beauty
In this everlasting light.

All the pain and grief is over,
Every restless tossing passed;
I am now at peace forever,
Safely home in Heaven at last.

Did you wonder I so calmly
Trod the valley of the shade?
Oh! But Jesus' love illumined
Every dark and fearful glade.

And He came Himself to meet me
In that way so hard to tread;
and with Jesus' arm to lean on
Could I have one doubt or dread?

Then you must not grieve so sorely,
For I love you dearly still;
Try to look beyond earth's shadows,
Pray to trust our Father's will.

There is work still waiting for you,
So you must not idly stand;
Do it now, while life remaineth-
You shall rest in Jesus' land.

When that work is all completed,
He will gently call you home;
Oh, the rapture of that meeting,
Oh, the joy to see you come!

Jeffrey's Obituary

God's Blessings

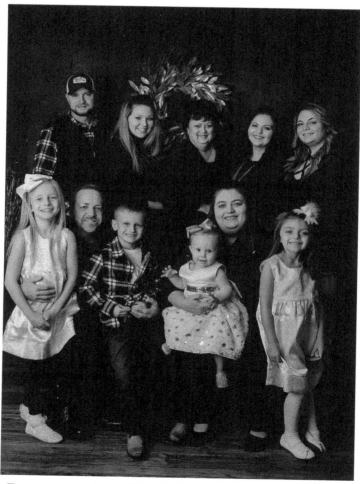

Front row: Madalyn, Billy, Parker, Maggie, Anita, Meredith.
Back row: Patrick, Lindsay, Linda, Megan, Lakin

CPSIA information can be obtained
at www.ICGtesting.com
Printed in the USA
BVHW090058240221
600894BV00019B/2325

9 781098 045357